Secrets Of A Healer - Magic of Hypnotherapy

SECRETS OF A
HEALER

VOL. VII
MAGIC OF HYPNOTHERAPY

Dr. Constance Santego

Maximillian Enterprises
Kelowna, BC

Secrets Of A Healer – Magic of Hypnotherapy
Copyright © 2020 by Dr. Constance Santego.

Copy Editor and Interior Design: Constance Santego
Book Layout: ©2017 BookDesignTemplates.com
Cover Design: Jennifer Louie

Ordering Information:
Quantity sales. Special discounts are available on quantity purchases by corporations, associations, and others. For details, contact the "Special Sales Department" at the address above.

Trade paperback ISBN: 978-0-9783005-9-3
Ebook ISBN 978-1-7770818-2-9
Created and published In Canada. Printed and bound in the United States of America

First Edition
Published by Maximillian Enterprises
Kelowna, BC
Canada
www.constancesantego.ca

Dedication

To My first Hypnotherapy Instructor, Sheldon.
You're in a deep....

Your Mind is where you will find all your Answers.

–Constance Santego

ALSO BY DR. CONSTANCE SANTEGO

FICTION
The Nine Spiritual Gifts Series:

Journey of a Soul – (Vol. 1 Michael)
Language of a Soul – (Vol. 2 Gabriel)
Prophecy of a Soul – (Vol. 3 Bath Kol)
Healing of a Soul – (Vol. 4 Raphael)

NON-FICTION
The Intuitive Life, The Gift of Prophecy, Third Edition

Fairy Tales, Dreams and Reality... Where Are You On Your Path?
Second Edition
Your Persona... The Mask You Wear
Angelic Lifestyle, A Vibrant Lifestyle
Angelic Lifestyle 42-Day Energy Cleanse
Archangel Michael's Soul Retrieval Guide

SECRETS OF A HEALER, SERIES:

Magic of Aromatherapy (Vol. I)
Magic of Reflexology (Vol. II)
Magic of The Gifts (Vol. III)
Magic of Muscle Testing (Vol. IV)
Magic of Iridology (Vol. V)
Magic of Massage (Vol. VI)
Magic of Hypnotherapy (Vol. VII)
Magic of Reiki (Vol. VIII)
Magic of Advanced Aromatherapy (Vol. IX)
Magic of Esthetics (Vol. X)

FOR CHILDREN

I am big tonight. I don't need the light!

Contents

Preface

The Miracle of Hypnotherapy

I was fourteen when my grandmother took me to see Reveen. I was mesmerized by his ability to put people into a trance state and suggest that they do something.

But it wasn't until I was in my thirties that I was hooked. I wanted to know how they did it! How did they make you do things that you said you couldn't do?

Once I found out that hypnosis was a type of meditation and that you were speaking directly to the subconscious mind is when I fell in love with it!

I have not found anything better than Hypnotherapy for helping a person be rid of their phobias, past hang-ups, fears, or self-sabotage acts.

I use a combination of Hypnotherapy with soooo many of the modalities I offer. It is one of the most incredible techniques I know how to do.

Note to Reader

Hypnotherapy *is not intended to replace traditional psychological techniques. Persons with deep psychological problems, extreme trauma, highly repressed memories should seek the service of a professional psychologist or therapist.*

Hypnotherapy is an excellent technique to use to for relaxation, stress-relief, clearing the mind, improve self-awareness, self-empowerment, and gaining laser-focus. You are ALWAYS in control of your situation, hypnosis has no power in healing you on its own, only you can do that.

Your Doctor still plays a vital role in your health care. If I break my leg, I will need a Doctor and all the nurses and staff that work in the Hospital.

Integrated Medicine focuses on that **we play** a significant role in taking care of our own health. What we put into our bodies, how hard we work our bodies, the stress level we allow into our everyday life, and the positive or negative energy we attract around us all play a role in our wellbeing. Shift happens...Create magic!

Learning Outcome

When you have completed this book and studied the concepts and techniques, you will be able to perform basic Hypnotherapy to help reduce stress, relax sore and achy muscles, and empower the body, mind, and soul. For you, your friends, and family.

- Relax, Rejuvenate, and Expand your Awareness,
- Learn the many Different Types of inductions and techniques,
- Bonus, learn how to perform the 'Energy Clearing Technique.'

PART ONE

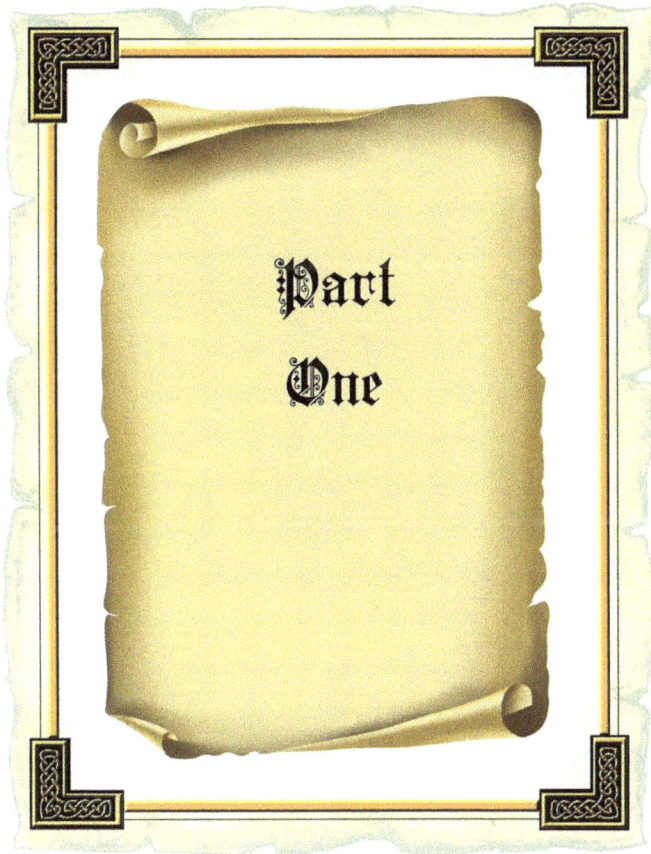

Part
One

What is Hypnotherapy?

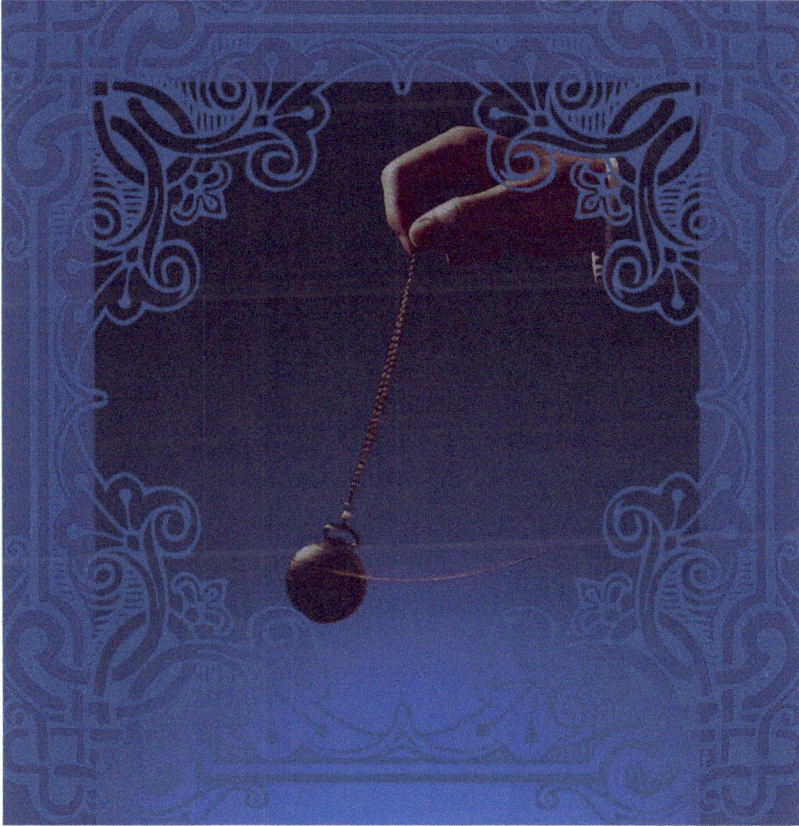

Oxford Definition of Hypnosis -the induction of a state of consciousness in which a person apparently loses the power of voluntary action and is highly responsive to suggestion or direction. It is used in therapy, typically to recover suppressed memories or to allow modification of behavior that has been revived but is still controversial.

Oxford Definition of Trance - a half-conscious state characterized by an absence of response to external stimuli, typically induced by hypnosis or entered by a medium.

OTHER DEFINITIONS

"Trance is channeling magnetic forces to attain equilibrium of invisible magnetic body fluid" (animal magnetism).

Franz Mesmer

"Trance is a lucid sleep."

James Braid

"Hypnosis is a means of communication ideas; a means of asking people to accept ideas and examine them, to discover the intrinsic meanings, and then to decide whether or not to act upon those particular meanings."

Milton Erickson

"Hypnosis or trance is the means to quiet the conscious mind (keep it busy), so we can access the subconscious and superconscious mind."

Constance Santego

Hypnotherapy vs Hypnosis

ypnotherapy is performed as a counseling technique, whereas hypnosis is performed as a stage act.

If you have ever gone to a magic show or hypnotic show, chances are you have witnessed hypnosis. Many famous magicians all know how to do hypnosis: Chris Angel, Derren Brown, and Peter Reveen, to name a few.

Stage Hypnosis is to entertain an audience. The Hypnotist performs anywhere from three to five pre-tests before choosing the participants. The Hypnotist is looking for people with specific traits, entertaining traits.

A hypnotist cannot make you do anything you would not do in real-life situations. This is why all the pre-tests, he needs people who are not under the influence of drugs or alcohol, too scared, are overthinking it, have mental issues, and just want to be hypnotized. The Hypnotist needs people who are not afraid to go on stage (not everyone gets up to go – filtering). He needs people who pass his tests.

Then once he has weeded out the beta people (who are not in an alpha state, which is the maximum brain activity needed), the Hypnotist can start with . . .

The first time I was hypnotized was in a bar, my sister and her friends wanted my husband and me to go with them. Once the Hypnotist asked the audience for people to come up on stage, my sister begged me to go up with her. I remember being squished between her and a guy. Preston was the Hypnotist at the time doing the show. He had us do a few pre-tests, like locking our hands together, then he came by and tested them to see if they broke apart. All I remember is feeling the guy's body heat leave (my eyes were closed) and my sisters.

Then Preston told us to pretend that we were playing an instrument that we had played in band class; I played the clarinet. That was easy. No harm was done. Then he kept putting us into a deep sleep, each time deeper than before. I must explain here that my children were two and three; sleep was a dream to me. To be honest, I stayed up on stage just to go to sleep. It was the best sleep I had ever had. I remember telling my husband that if I died, and that was Heaven, I was going to be in Bliss. He asked us to do nothing that I felt was embarrassing or immoral, so I stayed on stage, waiting to go back to sleep.

He had us take a break and return to our seats, but before we left the stage, he told us that when we get back, our friends and family would be speaking a rare Chinese language dialect, only known to a few people worldwide. I COULDN'T UNDERSTAND THEM once I got back to my seat with my family. I thought they were joking around. I finally turned my head into my husband's chest to ignore them, only to find they spoke English. As I turned around to tell them that it was not funny, they started to talk gibberish again. I was only too happy to get back on stage away from my crazy family.

Once Preston had finished with the act, he made a post-hypnotic suggestion. It was to enjoy life and prosper. Sitting back at my table, all my family was talking in English again.

Preston finished his act by having two big dudes from the audience come up on stage and sit on two chairs. They were facing away from each other. He put a coat on each back edge. Then he had a lady who he had kept on stage from our hypnosis group and told her she was a stiff, unbreakable, solid steel board. He had a couple of other guys from the audience help lift her onto the edges of the chairs, her neck on one edge and her ankles on the other. Her body was hovering above the ground, solid as a two-by-four. Preston brought over a third chair and climbed on top, then on top of her, and stood on her stomach. She barely flinched. I remember being amazed; she was a tiny person compared to him.

The other part that I was amazed at was what time it was. The show started at about 9:30 pm and was now 1:30 am! I was freaking out because I had told the babysitter we would be home at 11:00 pm (thank God it was a cousin of mine).

The Hypnosis show he performed ended up playing on our local T.V. channel for two years. It seemed everywhere I went. I had people telling me they saw me hypnotized on stage. The only good thing about it was I could watch the whole show (I didn't do anything I would have been embarrassed about, so all was good).

In Canada, well, B.C., for sure, you cannot perform stage hypnosis and be part of the counseling Hypnotherapy association. Hypnosis is strictly meant to help a person heal.

P.S. Being on stage, hypnotized, was nothing I thought it would be. I could hear everything the hypnotist was saying to everyone else, even with my eyes closed. Sleep is not what you think, and you are still conscious. I could have walked off that stage at any point, but he didn't do anything that I had a reason to. AND I wanted that sleep more than getting off the stage!!!

History of Hypnotherapy

Cuneiform writings date back to four thousand years before Christ reveals that Sumerians used Hypnosis as a therapeutic tool.

Specially trained **priest-doctors, Hindu fakirs, Persian magi,** and **Indian Yogi** gave hypnotic suggestions. **Ebers** papyrus says that ancient Egypt priest doctors had patients gaze at a shiny piece of metal (3000 BC, recorded on a stone stele).

There may be mention of Hypnosis in **the Bible** (Genesis 2:21, 1 Samuel 26:12, Job 4:13, 33:15, Acts 10:10) **Hippocrates** (430 BC) knew the importance of harmony between mind and body and described the mind as the 'seat of emotion.'

The **Ancient Egyptians** had their Temples of Sleep, and the **Greeks** had their Shrines of Healing, where patients were given curative suggestions while in induced sleep.

Franz Anton Mesmer (1734-1815) was an Austrian physician and a famed Medical School of Vienna graduate in 1776. He studied magnetism and used magnets to heal patients by passing them over the affected area while touching them with a metal rod. One day he was performing a session and had forgotten his magnets, he acted as if he had them, and to his surprise, the patient still healed. From that point on, he used his hands as his tool. Later, to Mesmer's request to prove his abilities to be true, He had three noteworthy men asses him. Benjamin Franklyn, one of those men, could not prove anything flowed from Mesmer's hands and said that he must be a Fraud and Mesmer was ruined.

In 1843 **James Braid** (1795-1860), a Scottish surgeon, termed 'hypnotism.' The name derives from 'Hypnos,' the Greek god of sleep. Braid coined the term expressly to discourage associating his hypnotic techniques with Mesmer's fanciful metaphysics.

1837, **John Elliotson,** Professor of Medicine at UCH, London, organized public clinical demonstrations of a wide range of hypnotic phenomena, exhibiting effects on voluntary and involuntary muscle, analgesia, somnambulism, hallucinations, etc., which he attributed to the magnetism theory. On his forced resignation, he edited a journal, The Zoist, in which he reported the work of James Esdaile, a Scottish surgeon was working in India who had performed several hundred operations relatively painlessly using hypnosis (mesmerism) alone as an anesthetic. He or an assistant would produce a state akin to suspended animation, now known as the Esdaile State, by stroking the patient's body for several hours. He recorded that fatal surgical shock or post-operative infection occurred in only 5% of cases compared with the then norm of 50%.

Sigmund Freud (May 6, 1856 – September 23, 1939) was an Austrian neurologist and the founder of the psychoanalytic school of psychology. He was referred to as 'the father of psychoanalysis.' Freud took up the study of medicine at Vienna; he studied neurology. Freud was big on hypnosis but spent most of his time on "free association."

Carl Gustav Jung (1875-1961) was the son of a Swiss pastor. He studied hypnotism in Zurich before becoming a devoted follower of Freud, a relationship that lasted from 1907 to 1913. Jung was Freud's favorite disciple. Jung's significance in clinical psychology, relative to Freud and the behaviorist B. F. Skinner, is minimal. Still, his influence - especially his idea of the "Collective Unconscious" - in New Paradigm and New Age thought and the popular mythology of the day is truly tremendous.

James Braid (1795 – March 25, 1860) coined the term and invented the procedure known as hypnotism. A surgeon, born in Fife, Scotland, and educated at the University of Edinburgh. Braid became interested in mesmerism when he observed demonstrations given by Charles Lafontaine. In 1843 he published Neurypnology: or the Rationale of Nervous Sleep, his first and only book-length exposition of his views. In this book, he coined the words hypnotism, hypnotize, and hypnotist, which remain in use—braid thought of hypnosis as producing a "nervous sleep," which differed from ordinary sleep. The most efficient way to produce it was through visual fixation on a small bright object held eighteen inches above and in front of the eyes. Braid regarded the physiological condition underlying hypnotism as the over-exercising of the eye muscles through the straining of attention.

Charles Lafontaine (1803 – 1892) was an early Swiss hypnotist. He lived in Geneva and published a journal called Le magnétiseur. He became wealthy as a traveling hypnotist or animal magnetizer, as it was then known. 1884 In Nancy, France, **Dr. Ambroise-August Liebeault** found that he could bring about cures in this state simply by suggestion.

Around this same time, **Jean Martin Charcot** was demonstrating his views at the Salpêtrière Hospital...that hypnosis was a pathological state akin to hysteria, the two phenomena being interchangeable.
In 1890 **Josef Breuer** and Sigmund Freud developed the application of hypnosis beyond the mere suggesting away of symptoms and changed the approach to the elimination of their apparent cause. Breuer found that in hypnosis, patients would often recall past events and, in talking about them, would experience an emotional outpouring, subsequently losing their symptoms. This he called his talking cure (we would now refer to this emotional state as an abreaction).

1914-18 During the Great War, the **Germans** realized that hypnosis was of value in the immediate treatment of shellshock, allowing soldiers to be returned rapidly to the trenches. A formularized version of hypnosis, autogenic training, was devised by a German, Dr. Schultz.
Dr. Orne's high profile and his term as President of the International Society of Hypnosis were instrumental in promoting hypnosis as a respected and respectable skill within psychology, medicine, and the legal field.

Milton H. Erickson, M.D., is considered the father of modern Hypnotherapy. The therapy he engendered, Ericksonian Hypnotherapy, is one of the fastest-growing and influential branches of Hypnotherapy today. His methods have inspired short-term strategic therapy, the rebirth of guided imagery, and NLP (Neuro-Linguistic Programming), to name a few. Erickson said, "Everyone is as individual as their thumbprint." In his practice, he tailored every induction to the person's individual needs and perceptual bias. He believed in the unconscious mind's wisdom and the theory that people have all the resources necessary to make changes inside themselves. He believed that the therapist's job is to help the person re-establish his or her connection with his or her inner resources and develop a rapport between the conscious and the unconscious mind. Often, Erickson didn't use a formal trance induction. Instead, he talks about stories that have a deeper meaning. Sometimes that meaning was clear; most times, it was not, at least not to the person's conscious mind.

Ernest Ropiequit Hilgard (1904-2001) was appointed Professor of Psychology at Stanford Ca in 1933. His major early interests were in learning and motivation, and two of his textbooks, Theory of Learning (1948) and Introduction to Psychology (1953) became classics. In 1957, he established the Stanford Laboratory of Hypnosis Research. Here he experimented with hypnotic pain reduction, and two books, Hypnosis in the Relief of Pain (1975) and Divided Consciousness (1977), became landmarks in the objective study of hypnosis. Hilgard further developed Janet's earlier work on dissociation into his theory of neo-dissociation, posing three stages of consciousness within hypnosis: the distorted reality, the hidden observer, and the observing consciousness.

John Hartland was a psychiatrist, a member of the BSMDH, and editor of the Journal of Medical Hypnosis. His comprehensive textbook on clinical Hypnotherapy, Medical & Dental Hypnosis was published in 1966. Hartland described straightforward techniques for ego and employing direct suggestions of a general nature to increase the patient's self-confidence. The book, now in its fourth edition, became a 'bible' for the medical or dental student of hypnosis.

Richard Bandler is a co-founder of John Grinder in Neuro-Linguistic Programming. A mathematics student, Richard began studying the work of Gestalt therapy founder Fritz Perls when he was asked to edit transcripts of Perls' lectures and workshops for the book "Eyewitness To Therapy" (1973) for Science and Behavior Books.

John Grinder Having graduated from the University of San Francisco (USF) with a degree in psychology in the early 1960s, Grinder studied Linguistics, for which he received his Ph.D. from the University of California at San Diego—drawing from the theory of transformational grammar, of the language patterns used by Gestalt Therapy founder Fritz Perls, family therapist Virginia Satir and Hypnotherapist Milton H. Erickson. Over the next three years, Grinder and Bandler continued to model these therapists' various cognitive behavioral patterns.

Canadian
Association of Co-operative Counselling Therapists
www.acctcounsellor.com

IACH -International Association of Counseling Hypnotherapists
www.Hypnotherapyassociation.org

United States
American Medical Association, 1958 – 1979 to present officially approved Hypnosis in medicine and dentistry.

Marc Savard, Stage Hypnosis school Las Vegas
http://www.marcsavard.net/hypnosisschool.html
The IACH does not recognize Stage Hypnosis. But if that is what you want to train for, Marc is one of the best.

Benefits

- Change negative behaviors, such as smoking, nail-biting, bed-wetting, and overeating
- Reduce fear, stress, and anxiety
- Eliminate or decrease the intensity of phobias
- Treat pain during childbirth and reduce labor time
- Control pain during dental and surgical procedures
- Relieve symptoms associated with irritable bowel syndrome (IBS)
- Lower blood pressure
- Lack of confidence
- Enhance creativity
- Exam/tests (nerves)
- Improve athletic performance
- Insomnia
- Motivation
- Sexual problems
- Teeth grinding
- Ulcers
- Negative energy
- Childhood issues
- Story Mode
- Past life regression (not covered by insurance)
- Control nausea and vomiting caused by chemotherapy
- Reduce the intensity or frequency of headaches, including migraines
- Treat and ease the symptoms of asthma
- Hasten the healing of some skin diseases, including warts, psoriasis, and dermatitis

Misconceptions

The Hypnotist is in control.

False: You are always in control during the hypnosis session. Hypnosis is a natural state you have experienced many times a day, for example, while watching TV, driving, reading a good book, at the movies, or concentrating very intently on a task.

Hypnosis is an altered state.

False: It is not. An altered state is your mind on LSD. Hypnosis is focused attention and a heightened sense of awareness.

I was not hypnotized if I heard and remembered everything about the session. I must be "out for the count."

False: You may hear and remember everything about your session. Hypnosis is a state of concentrated attention, so you are aware of the session.

You enter a hypnotic state by watching a swinging pendulum.

False: Not likely. Hypnotherapists typically give a person suggestions about mental and physical relaxation to help them reach the hypnotic state.

If I do not remember the hypnosis session, I was asleep and not hypnotized.

False: Some people experience such a profound state of relaxation that they may feel like they are asleep, but they are not. A hypnotist can periodically check during the session (for example, by having you signal with a finger) to ensure you are not asleep.

The Hypnotist can "make" me stop smoking, lose weight, etc.

False: Hypnosis is not magic, and a hypnotist cannot make a person do anything. The person must cooperate with the process.

The Hypnotist can make me do things I do not want to, like quacking like a duck.

False: A hypnotist cannot make you do anything, and you will reject any suggestion against your value system or beliefs.

The Hypnotist can find out things I do not want them to know about me.

False: Hypnosis is not a "truth serum," and you will not accidentally or otherwise reveal any secrets you do not want to.

I must see instant results, or the hypnosis didn't work.

False: The unconscious mind takes its time. Results may be seen at varying time intervals.

My problem should instantly go away with hypnosis.

False: It may take some time to work on your issue. Concentrate on any improvements, no matter how slight, in your issue.

I cannot be hypnotized.

False: Anyone of normal intelligence willing to follow instructions can be hypnotized. Of course, anyone can resist being hypnotized, also.

For hypnosis to work, I must reach a certain "depth" of trance.

False: Hypnosis can be effective whether you are in a light or deep trance.

Trance lets the conscious mind focus on one thing so the subconscious mind can bring to the surface more resources. Trance is like reading a great book or watching an awesome movie. After a few moments, you are in the story; trance is with even more intense realism.

Old School Procedure

The old-school belief was to have a script and follow it.

1-hour session

10 minutes

> Pre-induction talk
>
> What is the issue?
>
> What would they like out of the session?
>
> What would be the benefit, or what are they gaining?

15 -20 minutes

> Induction
>
> Progressive relaxation

5 -10 minutes

> Deepener
>
> Affirmations to the subconscious mind

10-15 minutes

> Teach what to do between sessions
>
> Build up the person's ego
>
> Bring the person out of the trance

5-10 minutes

> End the session

New School Procedure

The new school is to be spontaneous with the session and let the person lead.

1-hour session

5 - 10 minutes

Pre-induction talk

What is the issue?

Our job will be to have the person recognize the issue and find a way to release or change the emotions with the memory to a positive new thought.

5 -15 minutes

Induction and maybe deepening technique

15 - 40 minutes

- Have the person sense the issue:
- I have them go to an unusual place, like walking down a path, and along the path will be a building. They can enter the building.
- I have them go into the building and look around.
- This building will have a special room with an extremely comfortable chair for them to sit in and a big screen T.V or movie screen which is in front of them.
- They will use a remote control as you would on a Disc Player; rewind, fast forward, pause, or play and watch the scene as needed. The person can do this with no sound if they like. They can also zoom in or zoom out.

- I have them turn the Picture on and tell me what they see, hear, feel or think.
- *Whatever the answer is, I will write it down for later use. I might write down ten different things, depending on what they say.*
- When under hypnosis, I like to ask the person many questions: *these will be questions of what is to the point of the person's session, issues, outcome, etc.*

    o What are they seeing, feeling, thinking, and hearing?
    o How does this make them feel?
    o Where do they feel that in their body? (I would then do a color release from the meditation course).
    o What is the purpose of the issue?
    o What is the lesson?
    o Is there an easier way to fix this?
    o What have they learned in this session?

5-10 minutes (*Warn the person that the session will end in__?__ minutes.*)

End the session

Leslie M. LeCron & J. Bordeaux Scale

A guideline of phenomena that might occur during the different levels of trance.

SUSCEPTIBLE **DEPTH & SCORE**	SYMPTOMS AND PHENOMENA EXHIBITED
0	The subject fails to react in any way
HYPNOIDAL	
1	Physical relaxation
2	Drowsiness apparent
3	Fluttering of eyelids
4	Closing of eyes
5	Mental relaxation, partial lethargy of mind
6	Heaviness of limbs
LIGHT TRANCE	
7	Catalepsy of eyes
8	Partial limb catalepsy
9	Inhibition of small muscle group
10	Slower and deeper breathing, slower pulse
11	Strong lassitude (disinclination to move, speak, think or act)
12	Twitching of mouth or jaw during induction

13	The rapport between subject and operator
14	Simple post-hypnotic suggestions heeded
15	Involuntary start of eye
16	Personality changes
17	The feeling of heaviness throughout the entire body
18	The partial feeling of detachment
MEDIUM TRANCE	
19	Recognition of trance (difficult to describe but definitely felt)
20	Complete muscular inhibition (kinesthetic delusions)
21	Partial amnesia
22	Glove anesthesia
23	Tactile illusions
24	Gustatory illusions
25	Olfactory illusions
26	Hyperacuity of atmospheric conditions
27	Complete catalepsy of limbs/body
SOMNAMBULISTIC (SLEEPWALKING)	
28	Ability to open eyes without affecting trance

29	Fixed stare when eyes are open; papillary dilation
30	Somnambulism
31	Complete amnesia
32	Systematized post-hypnotic amnesia
33	Complete anesthesia
34	Post-hypnotic anesthesia
35	Bizarre post-hypnotic suggestions heeded
36	Uncontrolled movements of eyes; eye coordination lost
37	The sensation of lightness, floating, swinging, of being bloated, swollen, detached
38	Rigidity and lag in muscular movements and reactions
39	Fading and increase in cycles of the sound of the practitioner's voice (like the radio station fading in and out)
40	Control of organic body functions (heartbeat, blood pressure, digestion, etc.)
41	Recall of lost memories
42	Age regression

43	Positive visual hallucinations; post-hypnotic
DEPTH	
44	Negative visual hallucinations; post-hypnotic
45	Positive auditory hallucinations; post-hypnotic
46	Negative auditory hallucinations; post-hypnotic
47	Stimulation of dreams (in trance or post-hypnotic in natural sleep)
48	Hyper anesthesia
49	Color sensations experienced
50	Stuporous condition in which all spontaneous activity is inhibited.
SOMNAMBULISM	can be developed by suggestion to the effect

What Comes Next?

Basic Anatomy and Physiology of the Brain & Mind

CONSCIOUS, SUBCONSCIOUS, AND SUPERCONSCIOUS

THE BRAIN

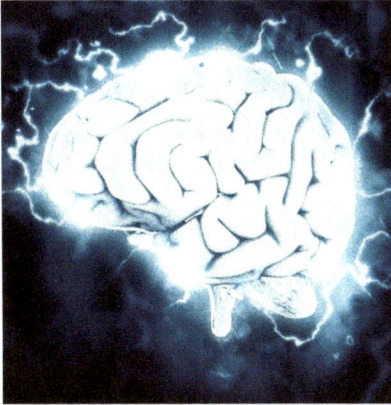

An organ of soft nervous tissue contained in the skull of vertebrates, functioning as the coordinating center of sensation and intellectual and nervous activity. Made up of the central nervous system (brain and spinal column)

CENTRAL NERVOUS SYSTEM (CNS) BRAIN AND SPINAL COLUMN

The brain is composed of three parts:
- the cerebrum (cerebral cortex) - consciousness,
- the cerebellum – unconscious,
- and the medulla oblongata - unconscious

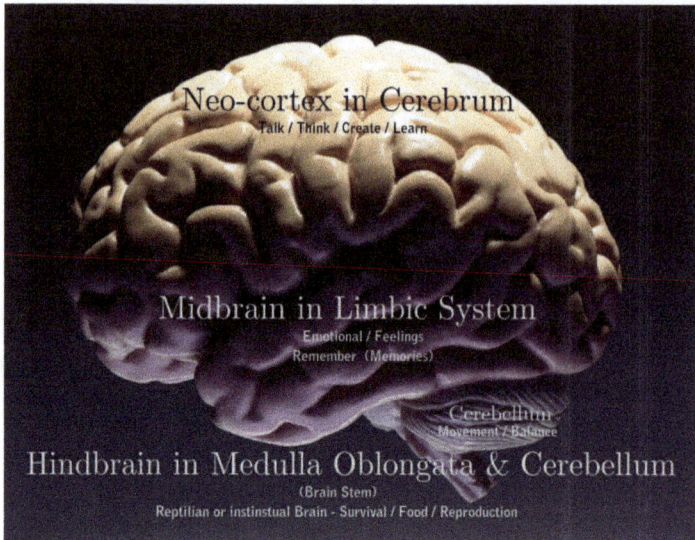

The 'Cerebrum' is the part of your brain that governs:

- intelligence
- learning
- reasoning
- memory
- personality
- behavior
- problem-solving
- emotional functions
- touch, vision, taste, hearing, smell, and the interpretation of spoken language, speech

You DO have 'Conscious' control, meaning you can change your actions.

The 'Cerebellum' is the part of the brain that governs:

All motor activity depends on the cerebellum.
- coordinate muscle movements,
- posture,
- reflexes
- and maintains equilibrium and balance

You DO NOT have 'Conscious' control, meaning you cannot change your actions. This part of your brain is subconscious.

The 'Medulla oblongata' is part of the brain that governs:

- breathing
- heartbeat
- movements of the eyes and mouth
- swallowing
- and sneezing

The function is to influence respiratory, cardiac, and vasomotor functions.

You DO NOT have 'Conscious' control, meaning you cannot change your actions. This part of your brain is subconscious.

Interesting Facts

The body will protect the brain more than any other part of the body. Your brain needs sugar to survive, whereas the rest of your body needs nutrients to survive.

The brain/blood barrier in your brain stops the blood from entering the brain while allowing other nutrients to enter.

The brain is like a computer. It has a basic function but needs to be programmed to do anything extra.

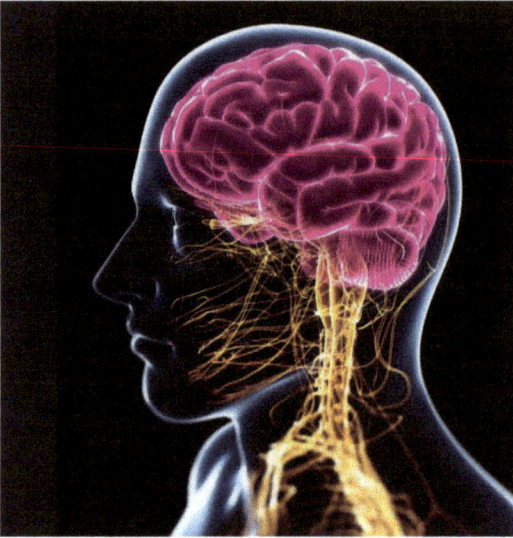

Your brain's electrical system is called the nervous system, consisting of the **Central Nervous System**- CNS, the supervisor of the body's nervous activity. Which is your **Brain, and the cord or tail runs** inside your **Spinal Column to your tailbone.**

And the Peripheral Nervous System- PNS, some sensory nerves, motor nerves, and both. These nerves extend from the brain and spinal cord BUT links the CNS to all other parts of the body (like your arms and legs).

Part of the PNS is the . . .

Somatic Nervous System (SNS)— the somatic nervous system is responsible for the voluntary control of skeletal MUSCLE and collecting SENSORY information from the body. The sensory information collected by the somatic nervous system arises from the skin and the musculoskeletal system. The information reaches our consciousness and is precisely mapped on the cerebral cortex.

Autonomic Nervous system— ANS, this system controls our organs. The ANS normally operates without voluntary (conscious) control. *Eg. When we climb stairs, our muscles are under conscious control and receive orders from the brain via the nerves of the PNS. But we are unaware of what our pancreas, liver, or spleen is doing while climbing.*

Two major divisions of the ANS:

> *Sympathetic—fight and flight*
> *Parasympathetic—rest and repair*

All systems in the body are important, BUT in Hypnotherapy, what we care about is the person's memories. Their BAD memories keep their dreams, wishes, wants and desires from becoming a reality.

As hypnotherapist our focus is on the 'Limbic System' of the brain, which is in the Cerebrum.

Close your eyes and imagine the center of your head. That is where the limbic system is.

LIMBIC SYSTEM

It is associated with emotions and feelings such as anger, sadness, sexual arousal, and pleasure. It is also associated with creativity, learning, and memory.

The three nervous system structures that make up the limbic system are the olfactory cortex (smell), the amygdala, and the hippocampus.

Olfactory cortex nerves directly connect your nose to the brain. Many associate a smell with an emotional issue (especially important in aromatherapy).

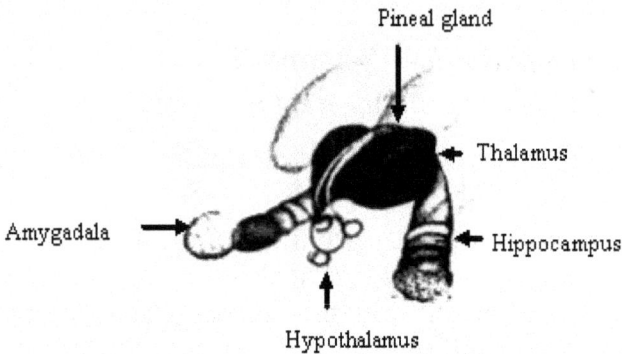

Amygdala

Two little almond-shaped structures (one in each brain hemisphere) connect with the hippocampus.

These connections make it possible for the amygdala to play an important role in mediating and controlling major affective activities like friendship, love and affection, on the expression of mood, and, mainly, fear, rage, and aggression.

The amygdala, the center for identifying danger, is fundamental for self-preservation. When triggered, it gives rise to fear and anxiety, leading the human into a stage of alertness, getting ready to fight or flight.

Experimental destruction of both amygdalas (there are two of them, one in each hemisphere) tames the animal, which becomes sexually non-discriminative, deprived of affection, and indifferent to danger. The electrical stimulus of these structures elicits crises of violent aggressivity.

Humans with marked amygdala lesions lose the affective meaning of the perception of outside information, like the sight of a well-known person. The subject knows precisely, who the person is, but cannot decide whether he likes or dislikes him (or her).

Hippocampus

It is particularly involved with MEMORY phenomena, especially with forming long-term memory (the one that sometimes lasts forever).

Nothing can be retained in the memory when both hippocampi (right and left) are destroyed. The subject quickly forgets any recently received message. The intact hippocampus allows the human to compare the conditions of a present threat with similar past experiences, thus enabling it to choose the best option to guarantee its survival.

The Hypothalamus and Thalamus (endocrine system)

Lesions of the hypothalamic nuclei interfere with several vegetative functions and some of the so-called motivated behaviors, like thermal regulation, sexuality, combativeness, hunger, and thirst.

The hypothalamus is also believed to play a role in emotion. Specifically, its lateral parts seem to be involved with pleasure and rage, while the median part is like to be involved with aversion, displeasure, and a tendency to uncontrollable and loud laughing.

However, in general terms, the hypothalamus has more to do with emotion expression (symptomatic manifestations) than with the genesis of the affective states.

When the physical symptoms of emotion appear, the threat they pose returns, via the hypothalamus, to the limbic centers and, thence, to the pre-frontal nuclei, increasing anxiety. This negative feedback mechanism can be so strong as to generate a situation of panic. As will be seen later, the knowledge of this phenomenon is especially important for clinical and therapeutic reasons. Imagine the amygdala is the antenna sensing danger, and the hippocampus is the receiver that relays the message to the hypothalamus, which is the transmitter and relays it to the pituitary, which forwards it to the appropriate gland, which stimulates a reaction in the body.
How I like to explain the role of the mind is this, imagine the Hypothalamus as the government. It makes up all the rules.

The pituitary is the general of the army. And all the other glands in the body are the army's privates. When the government (hypothalamus gland) gives an order to the general (pituitary gland), the general relay the directions to his army (all the other endocrine glands), which follow orders, and the action of intent is performed.

Your memories are stored now, depending on how good or bad they are! Your mind only keeps the best or worst thoughts and turns them into memories. BUT this sorting of thoughts happens at night when you are sleeping and unconscious!!!

Your limbic system sorts your thoughts, tosses out the mediocre ones, and only keeps the most emotional experiences. In a Hypnotherapy trance state, you can only recall your best or worst memories, nothing in between.

The limbic system does this by filtering your thoughts. In your sleep, when all your conscious functions are sleeping. Both the left and right amygdala evaluate and sort all your thoughts into categories of importance. The amygdala tells your brain if you need to fight or flight (run away). Part of the brain decides if what you felt today was a threat and keeps the memory in case you need to be reminded to run later.

Memory

- The faculty by which the mind stores and remembers information.

We remember things by association. All information in our memory is associated with another.

Think of an orange; color, texture, shape, smell, taste, fruit, and nutrients. We do not think of an elephant when thinking of an orange unless there is some interesting story to the thought (I bet you also now have a thought or image of an elephant).

Most of us have a good memory, but we don't have practice in using it efficiently.

Two things must happen to remember something:

1st, you need to be in the same state of awareness. If we arrive home from work exhausted, hungry, carrying bags or paperwork, telling the kids to do their homework, and tripping over the dog while kicking off our shoes, it is no wonder that our keys are missing in the morning.

2nd, you need a destination/location for your keys, no matter what you do. Be it your purse, tabletop, key hanger, etc. In the morning, you are in a different state of consciousness, usually refreshed and ready to go (unless you did not get your coffee –which is another memory stimulus – caffeine and habit)

You can improve your memory by forming associations or habits with what is important to you. A habit takes twenty-one days to develop or break, and sometimes it needs a refresher months later. Depending on how long the habit has been practiced.

MRI

Magnetic Resonance Imaging brain scans have shown that women have up to sixteen areas of the brain to evaluate others' behavior, and men have up to six.

Women's brains are designed more for multi-tasking than men's. However, anyone can develop their brain to recognize minimal cues or multitask.

You can store something to memory by repetition, like when you learned you're A, B, or C's (long-term memory) or for a test (short-term memory). The hippocampus is the part of your brain that controls long and short-term memory.

THE MIND

The element of a person that enables them to be aware of the world and their experiences, to think, and to feel; is the faculty of consciousness and thought.

We can take a picture of your brain, but not your mind.

SOMETHING INTERESTING FOR YOUR MIND

Read the note below...You will be amazed...

The paomnnehil pweor of the hmuan mnid.
Aoccrdnig to a rscheearch at Cmabrigde Uinervtisy, it deosn't mttaer in waht oredr the
ltteers in a wrod are, the olny iprmoetnt tinhg is taht the fist and lsat ltteer be at the rghit
pclae. The rset can be a taotl mses and you can sitll raed it wouthit porbelm. This is
bcuseae the huanm mnid deos not raed ervey lteter by istlef, but the wrod as a wlohe.

AMZANIG HUH?

Conscious Mind:

- The state of being aware of and responsive to one's surroundings.
- Stored in the *amygdale (limbic system)*
- Acts as a filter for thought or outside influences.
- Thinks or analyzes information
- Controls our movements
- Responsibilities
- 7 to 9,000,000,000.00 bits of information every second. We only consciously notice about 9 bits.
- In seconds:
  - From sight to touch 0.071
  - From touch to sight. 0.053
  - From sight to hearing 0.16
  - From hearing to sight 0.06
  - From one ear to another 0.064

Subconscious Mind

- Of or concerning the part of the mind of which one is not fully aware but which influences one's actions and feelings.
- Stored in ***the hippocampus (limbic system)***
- Stores your belief system, self-image, morals, habits, emotions, fears, secrets, and memories
- Cannot tell the difference between real or imagined
- Understands subliminal messages
- Ability to solve problems creatively
- Dreams
- Some believe Psychic ability is accessed here

Superconscious Mind

- Transcending human or normal consciousness: Universal mind of God:
- Higher self.
- Accessible through Meditation, yoga breathing, and hypnosis
- Group consciousness or God consciousness
- Healing
- All knowing
- Akasha records can be obtained
- Brilliant ideas, music, art, movies, stories, and concepts are formatted here- Einstein, Nostradamus, etc.

Levels of Consciousness

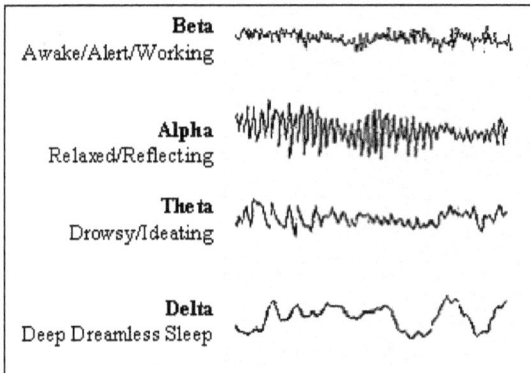

Beta Awake/Alert/Working	~~~~~~~
Alpha Relaxed/Reflecting	~~~~~~~
Theta Drowsy/Ideating	~~~~~~~
Delta Deep Dreamless Sleep	~~~~~~~

Scientists have found that our brain operates in four frequency levels: beta, alpha, theta, and delta, and each frequency (hertz) is measured in cycles per second.

The electroencephalograph (EEG) is a machine that monitors brainwave activity.

Beta- 11-40 C.P.S. (Hertz - C.P.S.=cycles per second)
(higher the number higher the stress level)

- Conscious (awake)
- Normal waking state
- Active conversation
- Speech
- Teacher
- Talk show host
- Problem-solving
- Doing
- Logical thinking
- Analysis
- Active attention

Alpha - 8-11 C.P.S.

- Subconscious
- Daydreaming
- Deeply relaxed
- Meditation
- Inspiration
- Fantasizing
- Creative visualization
- Completed task

When awake, you fluctuate between beta (doing something), and alpha (meditative) states all day.

The following two levels are during your sleeping state.

Theta - 3 ½ - 8 C.P.S.
- Subconscious
- Dream sleep
- Learning facts
- Imagination
- Ideas
- Creative thinking
- Highway driving
- Automatic tasks – showering/brushing teeth
- Intuition
- Deep meditation
- Dominant state for children 2 to 5

Delta - ½ -3 ½ C.P.S.
- Unconscious
- Dreamless sleep
- Deep sleep (approximately 2 hours each night)
- Body Heals
- Soul regenerates

Brain Dead- 0 C.P.S.

When you are in bed reading, you are in the Beta state. Turn the lights out and close your eyes. You will start in the Alpha state (conscious dreaming), moving into Theta (dreaming -dream cycle is about ninety-minute cycles, REM-rapid eye movement) and Delta throughout the night.

For Hypnotherapy, the Alpha state is usually the state
you want your person to be in, relaxed and able to
communicate with you.

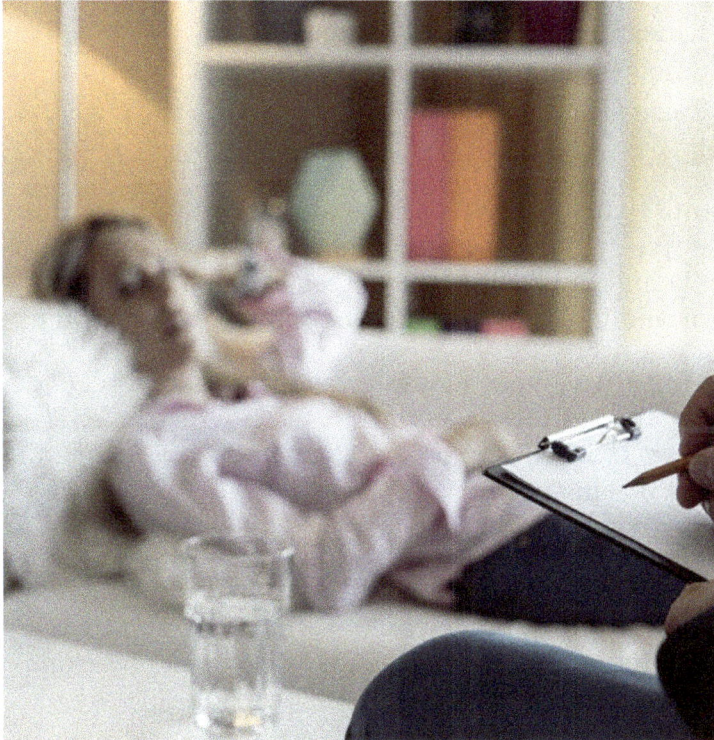

Holistic Counseling

Humans communicate through five proven senses:

- Vision
- Auditory (sound)
- Kinesthetic (touch and emotion)
- Smell (Olfactory)
- Taste (Gustatory)

A person's external environment stimulates one or more of these five senses. Then the information is taken internally and fed back to the external world through behavior and language through the same sensory system.

Interesting note – your memories are stored and related mainly by the sensory system it was received by. AND the sensory system, which a person is most aware of and uses most often, is the primary one.

This knowledge will help determine how to release the memory for a Hypnotherapist. If there were a distinct smell in the memory, you would want the person to activate (remember) the scent and release the emotions simultaneously with the smell.

REMEMBER to ask these questions; what are you Seeing? Hearing? Feeling? Smelling? Tasting?

Body Language

As a Hypnotherapist, you will need to start noticing the person's body language. These subtle changes will tell you more of the truth about how the person feels than the person might.

- Posture
- Movement
- Twitches
- Muscle tension
- Facial expressions
- Breathing – rate, pauses, location, volume
- Skin color
- Lip size, color
- Pupil dilation
- Tone and volume of voice
- Speed, tempo
- Intonation
- Location of voice in the body

Go to a public place and start people-watching, a mall, amusement park, café, a bench in a park, or at the beach. Anywhere and everywhere, start reading people.

—

An excellent book to read 'The Definitive Book of Body Language.' And an excellent series to watch is, 'Lie to Me.'

- Crossed legs and arms means in defense mode
- Fidgety or fast words mean nervous
- Stumbling words or forgets means they are probably close to the truth.

EYE MOVEMENT

From my book "Your Persons...The Mask You Wear"

On average, we are all born with the same basic neurology. We learn to walk, talk, play, work, etc.. How we do this is due to our nervous system. We do this well due to our upbringing (culture) and beliefs (personal and society).

Their right...Your left   *Their left...Your right*

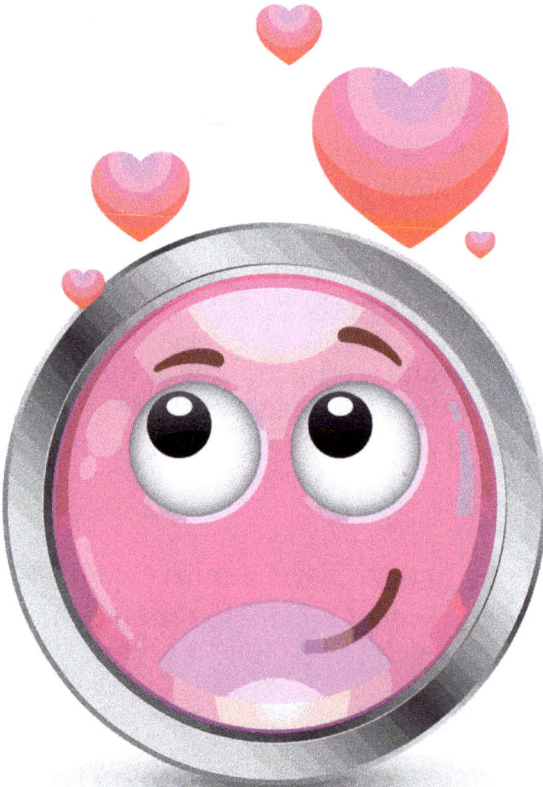

EYE ACCESSING CHART

As if you are looking at a person or a mirror.

<u>Their right, your left</u>
<u>Their left, your right</u>

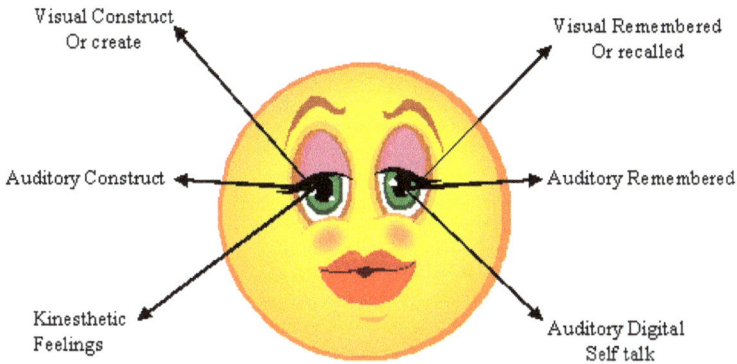

Visual Construct
Or create

Visual Remembered
Or recalled

Auditory Construct

Auditory Remembered

Kinesthetic
Feelings

Auditory Digital
Self talk

*I have found that a look
straight at you is Knowing*

Which direction are the eyes facing?

Meanings of the direction of eye movements:

Visuals will look like this when asked a question:

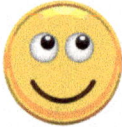

Visual Remembered
- the person is remembering a visual memory

Looking up to their left (your right)

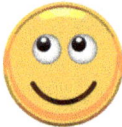

Visual Constructed
- the person is creating a visual image
(not real, they are making it up, great for meditation or hypnosis)

Looking up to their right (your left)

Audios will look like this when asked a question:

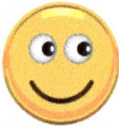

Auditory Remembered
- the person is remembering hearing a memory

Looking across to their left (your right)

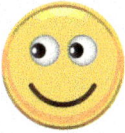

Auditory Constructed
- the person is creating hearing a sound
(not real, they are making it up)

Looking across to their right (your left)

Feelers will look like this when asked a question:

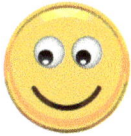

Kinesthetic
- the person is feeling a memory

Looking down to their right (your left)

Knowers will look like this when asked a question:

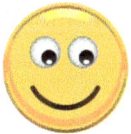

Self-talk
- Can be a sign for Knower
- The person is usually repeating in their mind what you just said.

Looking down to their left (your right)

*This next one was not taught in the NLP course; this is just what I found when studying my students:

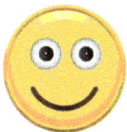

Knowing
- the person is remembering a fact

Looking straight at you

SOME QUESTIONS TO ASK
TO TEST THEIR EYE MOVEMENTS:

A person may do more than one eye movement with any one question.

Subconsciously the first place they look is always their first channel. But once they consciously think about the question, their eyes will change direction.

Ask the questions, but watch where the person's eyes are moving, or use a second person to watch while you read.

<u>Some Visual Channel Questions:</u>

Visual remembered

>What color is _____?

>What does _____ look like?

>Can you see _____?

Visual Constructed

>Can you imagine the view from the moon?

>What color would you like your next car to be?

>Can you imagine the bottom half of _____ with the top half of _____?

Some Audio Channel Questions:

Audio remembered

Can you hear _____?

Can you recall the sound of _____?

What is something you say to yourself?

Audio constructed

Can you hear the sound of _____ changing into _____?

Combine the sound of _____ with _____?

Can you hear the sound of ____ and _____ at the same time?

Some Feeler Channel Questions:

Feeler

Can you recall the feeling of _____?

How does _____ feel to you?

Do you feel the sensation of _____?

Some Knower Channel Questions:

Knower

Any of the questions... but usually, they instantly answer and never blink or look away. They look straight at you, or they may look down to the right.

BODY MOVEMENT

People's body movements will also tell you the same as their eyes.

If a person's hand(s) move out

- To their sides = audio
- Up around their shoulders or head = visual
- Lower or hip area = feeler
- Straight ahead = knower.

Leg movements, foot movements, and head tilting can give you more hints about their main channel.

Example: You are conversing with a friend, and you ask them this question.

"Tell me about your childhood."

Also, watch what happens to their body movements. Okay, if all that moved were their eyes (go to the NLP chart). But sometimes a person starts to talk with their body, hands or feet move, or they start to fidget side to side.

- Did they stare at you and not move a muscle when answering your question, or did they ask you what you wanted to know?
  Knower trait

- Did they start moving their right or left foot while talking to you?
  Their Left is self-talk (our right – means they are re-saying what you just said in their head).
  Any one of the channels may do this.

Usually a Knower trait.

Their Right is a <u>Feeler</u> trait *(our left),* meaning they returned to the emotions of being a kid.

- Did they talk with a hand to the sides of their body?

   Left or Right is an <u>Audio</u> trait

- Did they tilt their head up to one side while talking?

   Left or Right is a <u>Visual</u> trait

There is nothing wrong if they are doing a combination of the movements. It just means this will not be an easy test to decide which personality channel they are.

Hypnotherapy Counseling Rules for the Practitioner

Take notice of what people joke about, it may be the truth!

CONFIDENTIALITY

All information is NOT to be discussed with anyone without written consent from the person. Confidentiality is a must with the person's session or written information. Please do not talk to anyone other than the person about their session unless the person has given a written release form. Other than being subpoenaed by court order.

AVOID PANIC

Keep your voice soft and in control. Literal words are especially important. We should not panic, misinterpret, or try to artificially or dutifully change our reactions or other people's.

THE THREE RULES

1. If a person speaks about suicide,
2. hurting someone or themselves,
3. or anything bad or immoral with a child,

You MUST tell the authorities (Police, social services, etc.) about it.

EYE CONTACT

Always maintain eye contact, BUT only if the person likes eye contact.

ENDINGS

Choices on how to end a session:

- Always tell the person ahead of time:
    1. You have (e.g., Ten) minutes left for us to finish up this session
    2. We have (e.g., Ten) minutes left to finish the session, and we will continue the next session.
- Always make sure the person has something positive to go with. Ask them to tell you what the positive is.

HOSTILE PERSONS

If you have a person who is getting mad, simply acknowledge the emotion.

I have noticed this seems to bring up an angry (or another emotion) feeling in you when you talk about this.

Where in your body do you feel this?

Ask the person if they would like to release this.

If 'Yes,' then have the person breathe this feeling out. You may put color to it and then change it to their favorite color.

REFUSAL TO HYPNOTHERAPY

A person may refuse at any time to terminate the session!

You will refuse to hypnotize anyone:

- Under the influence of alcohol or drugs,
- With a mental disorder,
- Wanting to work on their childhood issues,
- Under the legal age (you need a degree for that).

Simply advise the person that Hypnotherapy cannot be provided without a physician's written approval.

UNDER NO CIRCUMSTANCES CAN A PERSON FORCE YOU TO PROVIDE A SESSION IF YOU FEEL IT IS UNSAFE.

PERSON/PRACTITIONER BOUNDARIES

- Person Neglect
  - o Unintentional physical or emotional harm resulting from practitioner insensitivity or lack of knowledge.
- Person Abuse
  - o Physical or emotional harm sustained from deliberate acts of the practitioner
- Boundaries are best established and maintained through communication
- Confidentiality is a must with the person's session or written information. Please do not talk to anyone other than the person about their session. Unless the person has given a written release form. Other than being subpoenaed by court order.
- Person safety is a must! Physically and Emotionally
- Intellectual boundaries
  - o Beliefs, thoughts, and ideas
- Financial boundaries
  - o The price of a session will always be told and agreed upon before a session
- A mistake many practitioners make is becoming a friend of the person. Business should stay business, and if a friendship develops outside of the massage room, then have the new friend go to someone else.
- If an intimate relationship should develop...it is said that six months of discontinuing the person-practitioner relationship before the new relationship is initiated.
- Even flirting is considered sexual misconduct and is not permitted.
- Selling products to a person is a conflict of interest. If you have products, they may be displayed outside the massage room and never be implied they must buy, only suggested they could buy. It should be similar to a store, where a person

may browse and look but not need to buy anything else.

COUNSELING SKILLS

Pre-Session:
- Tell them up front your time, place, duration, and price,
- How to get to the office,
- May want to have 20 min- ½ hour assessment session.
- One hr. sessions – (2 hrs. are exceptionally long and tiring for both practitioner and the person),
- Be careful of the person making an appointment right after a session with you. Have the person call you the next day to make the next appointment (people can be very vulnerable when under stress),
- Interruptions- phones, noises, etc. Do not have any!
- The counseling room does not have many talk pieces, photos, models, etc.

HELPING PRINCIPALS

In holistic counseling, you will need to know a few rules.

1. It is important that it is the person who makes the appointment with you, not someone else.
2. The person is in control of their emotional investment and involvement in their healing
3. We must be in a friendly relationship with the person we assist. It helps if we like them
4. Do not try to have every person like you.
5. Keep the session about the person!
6. Sitting Arrangements
   a. When a practitioner sits behind a desk— they may say that they need to protect themselves or to impress a person (big boss). Sit sideways to the person.
7. Do not ever take the person's power. Instead, empower them –when the person is in control, they are empowered.
8. The Person is to find the answers. We do not give our opinion
9. Do not try to process them for your ego
10. Take ourselves and our reactions into account at the same time. We must know what is taking place within ourselves and with them simultaneously. We do not counsel ourselves on their time. The session is for them!!!
11. We need to be able to relate *a bit* to understand what the person's words, motions, etc., mean.
12. We do not have to solve problems; we only must help the other person accept that responsibility for themselves
13. We need to listen
14. We only give others our time, understanding, and our honest selves, nothing else.

15. Good counseling demands less and more, at the same time, less concern about us and more humanity about them.
16. Counselors who can let go of themselves lessen the demand on themselves.
17. Let the person pause and absorb what they have been able to discover about themselves
18. Support the person when they enter the experience of exploring themselves
19. Do not judge others
20. Just be yourself; empathetic, flow, intent, and honest

PRACTITIONERS POSITION AND SPEECH

Be trustworthy and honorable!

Respecting the person, regardless of the method or approach you choose with a particular person, is extremely important to respect and honor the subject's integrity and beliefs. A student or practitioner should never attempt to impose their beliefs on anyone. Working within the belief system of the subject is always more effective. The premise is that a partnership is developing. You are working together to create the experience of the subject choice.

Seating position: You want the person to feel as safe and comfortable as possible. Many practitioners use a lazy boy chair for their persons to relax in. A bed is too much like sleeping, and you do not want your person to go to sleep in a trance.

Your chair should be to the side of your person, where your legs point to the side of your person and not directly at them. The straight-on position is very intimidating and will cause uneasiness.

Some methods of developing Trust:
- Mirroring – copying the movements of the person
- Empathy – Feeling and demonstrating concern
- Pacing – Timing your breath or any other observed rhythmic movement to the person's

- Language – Use the person's way of speaking (wording)
- Voice Inflection – Be aware of the tone of your voice. Breathe deeply & slowly
- Attitude –
  - Relax.
  - Demonstrate confidence.
  - Do not put yourself in a superior position to the person.
  - Relate at the same level.
  - Maintain an attitude of curiosity.

Speech should be relaxed and congruent with what the practitioner is saying. It always has rhythm and flows smoothly. Choppy sentences can create tension. Your speed of talking should go with what you are describing. Many Hypnotherapists have a special tone of voice when talking to a person in a trance. It is their trance voice and never monotones in sound.

Your tone of voice will produce a vibration that relaxes or irritates the person. Some students are naturally inducing trance, and others need practice. If you need practice, make sure you try different tones of the tone of voice when inducing a trance.

Choice of words is to the practitioner's style and, most importantly, the person's personality and belief system. You may have to change your person's style. Speak at the person's breathing or a bit slower (if you want them to relax even more).
Word choice: (use with a person)

- Descriptive words:
- Sense words: color, texture, sounds, tastes, and smells
- Repeating words: person retains information
- Permissive suggestions: in a moment, you will..., perhaps...either one or the other...
- Direct suggestions: you will..., turn to your left..., the forest is peaceful...
- Indirect suggestion: storytelling and visualization...
- Subliminal: unobtrusive gesture, change of pitch, glance away
- Use conjunctions: *and, but, if,* or casual words: *since..., and because...*

Your person will take every word you say to the extreme literal meaning. Be very careful with what words you use. You may say see or visualize, and your person can not easily do that, so use the word 'sense' or 'imagine'.

When giving suggestions, use positive words instead of negative words. '**Do not or don't** eat cake'... rather, say, "You choose to eat healthily."

Remember, the subconscious mind is very literal when information is received. Every word, affirmation, and suggestion is extremely important.

- Do not use negative or negative reinforcement unless for a specific purpose in rare circumstances.
- Do not use any suggestion that creates undue stress
- Do not use any suggestion to eliminate pain unless it is for a specific condition. Then only under the supervision of a Medical Doctor.

- Through suggestion, create an attitude that the person has already succeeded.
- All suggestions must be lawful, logical, and reasonable to the person.
- Always inform the person what suggestions you will use and get their permission.
- Always cancel any suggestion in which there is no need for a post-induction effect.

Ensure you know what your person is afraid of so that you never use images or ideas. I give my person's choice many times.

MASLOW'S HIERARCHY OF NEEDS

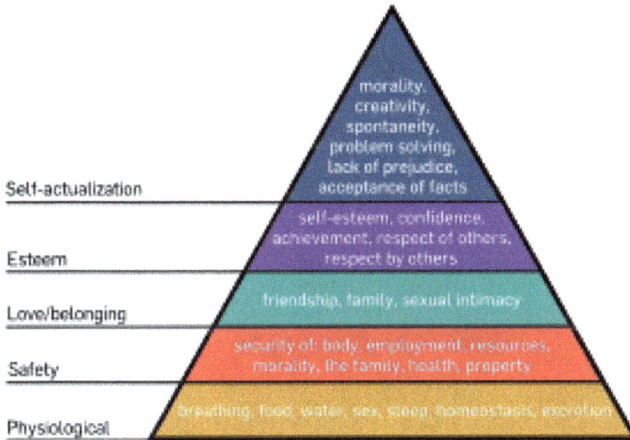

Mazlow's Hierarchy of Needs

In order of importance, this diagram represents the basic needs of a human being. You cannot help someone whose basic needs are not being met.

If the person comes to you to improve their self-esteem and they have nowhere to sleep, you will not be able to help them until they have a place to sleep.

As long as your person's physiological and safety are okay, you can proceed to have them choose an area in their life they would like to improve:

- Family
- Personal Growth
- Relationships
- Job or Career
- Health & Fitness
- Spirituality

Ask the person or have them write it down:

- What is important to them?
- How will your present behaviors and beliefs affect your goal (values)? Have the person write them out and number them in importance.
- What is important?
- Why are these important?
- What stops you from having more of it?
- What stops you from having it now?
- What do you feel when you don't achieve your goal (Fears & Beliefs)?
- What you will get from achieving your goal.

In Canada, the counseling guidelines are written in the book 'Choices.'

Textbook– Choices, Interviewing and Counselling Skills for Canadians ISBN 0130665851

Tidbit of knowledge- counseling is the English spelling, and counseling is the United States spelling.

FEELINGS INVENTORY

The following are words we use to express emotional states and physical sensations. This list is neither exhaustive nor definitive. It is meant as a starting place to support anyone who wishes to engage in deepening self-discovery and facilitate greater understanding and connection between people.

There are two parts to this list: feelings we may have when our needs **are** being met and feelings we may have when our needs are **not** being met.

The contents of this page can be downloaded and copied by anyone so long as they credit CNVC as follows:

(c) 2005 by the Center for Nonviolent Communication
Website: www.cnvc.org

Feelings when your needs are satisfied

AFFECTIONATE
compassionate
friendly
loving
open-hearted
sympathetic
tender
warm

CONFIDENT
empowered
open
proud
safe
secure

ENGAGED
absorbed
alert
curious
engrossed
enchanted
entranced
fascinated
interested
intrigued
involved
spellbound
stimulated

INSPIRED
amazed
awed
wonder

EXCITED
amazed
animated
ardent
aroused
astonished
dazzled
eager
energetic
enthusiastic
giddy
invigorated
lively
passionate
surprised

EXHILARATED
blissful
ecstatic
elated
enthralled
exuberant
radiant
rapturous
thrilled

GRATEFUL
appreciative
moved
thankful
touched

HOPEFUL
expectant
encouraged
optimistic

JOYFUL
amused
delighted
glad
happy
jubilant
pleased
tickled

PEACEFUL
calm
clear-headed
comfortable
centered
content
equanimous
fulfilled
mellow
quiet
relaxed
relieved
satisfied
serene
still
tranquil
trusting

REFRESHED
enlivened
rejuvenated
renewed
rested
restored
revived

Feelings when your needs are <u>not</u> satisfied

AFRAID
apprehensive
dread
foreboding
frightened
mistrustful
panicked
petrified
scared
suspicious
terrified
wary
worried

ANNOYED
aggravated
dismayed
disgruntled
displeased
exasperated
frustrated
impatient
irritated
irked

ANGRY
enraged
furious
incensed
indignant
irate
livid
outraged
resentful

DISCONNECTED
alienated
aloof
apathetic
bored
cold
detached
distant
distracted
indifferent
numb
removed
uninterested
withdrawn

DISQUIET
agitated
alarmed
discombobulated
disconcerted
disturbed
perturbed
rattled
restless
shocked
startled
surprised
troubled
turbulent
turmoil
uncomfortable
uneasy
unnerved
unsettled
upset

PAIN
agony
anguished
bereaved
devastated
grief
heartbroken
hurt
lonely
miserable
regretful
remorseful

SAD
depressed
dejected
despair
despondent
disappointed
discouraged
disheartened
forlorn
gloomy
heavy-hearted
hopeless
melancholy
unhappy
wretched

AVERSION
animosity
appalled
contempt
disgusted
dislike
hate
horrified
hostile
repulsed

CONFUSED
ambivalent
baffled
bewildered
dazed
hesitant
lost
mystified
perplexed
puzzled
torn

EMBARRASSED
ashamed
chagrined
flustered
guilty
mortified
self-conscious

FATIGUE
beat
burnt out
depleted
exhausted
lethargic
listless
sleepy
tired
weary
worn out

TENSE
anxious
cranky
distressed
distraught
edgy
fidgety
frazzled
irritable
jittery
nervous
overwhelmed
restless
stressed out

VULNERABLE
fragile
guarded
helpless
insecure
leery
reserved
sensitive
shaky

YEARNING
envious
jealous
longing
nostalgic
pining
wistful

PART TWO

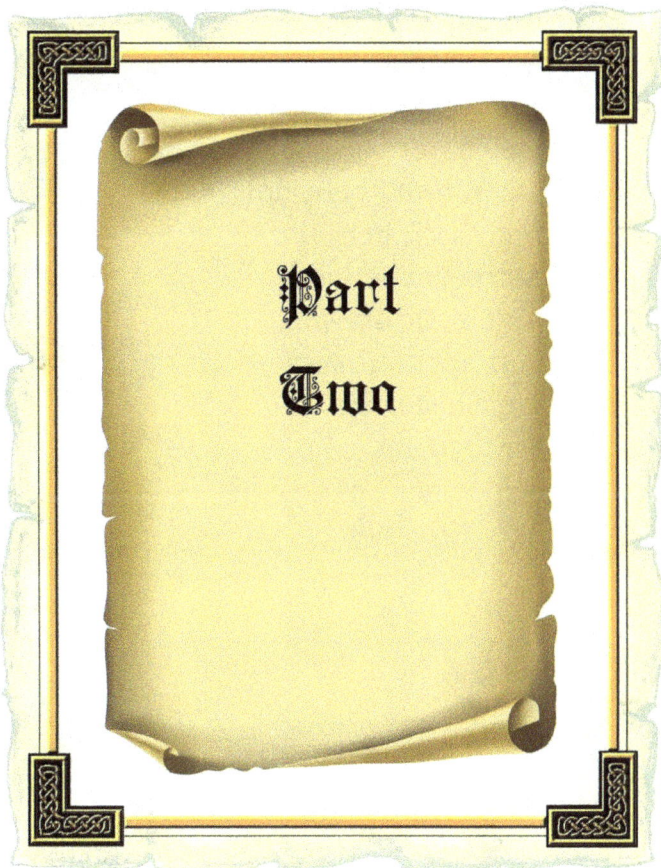

CLASSIC HYPNOTIC PHENOMENON

- Hallucinations
- Positive
- Negative
- Anesthesia
- Analgesic
- Catalepsy
- Ideomotor behavior
- Ideosensory behavior
- Automatic behavior
- Automatic writing
- Automatic drawing
- Post hypnotic suggestion
- Time distortion
- Amnesia
- Hyper amnesia
- Age regression

SIGNS OF BEING IN A TRANCE

Some people may not feel hypnotized because they can hear, move, open their eyes, get up if they want to, think, talk, or move. Here are some of the signs of being in a trance:

- Body temperature changes, usually cooler
- Fluttering of eyes
- Redding of the eyes (relaxation causes the blood to flow)
- Eyes may start to water
- Eyes may have rapid eye movement (REM)
- Eyes rollback
- Slower breathing
- Slower talking, quieter, and less annunciated
- Stomach noises
- More lethargic
- Dissociation
- Facial or body movements may react to comments
- Pleasant tingling in arms and or legs
- A feeling of heaviness or lightness or relaxed
- Hands/arms/legs feel like they are not there
- The chair and you feel like one
- Reluctance to move
- Time distortion (feels like minutes, not an hour)
- Rested
- Outside noises intensify (make sure you have the person focus on your voice)
- Heaviness in muscles
- Floating feeling
- Twitching

ABREACTIONS

This is when a person's response in the hypnotic state is unexpected and usually occurs spontaneously.

Examples:

Eyes open suddenly in the trance

This sometimes happens when the person is in a trance, usually the first time. The person opens their eyes to reassure themselves.

Carry on the session.

RESISTANCE TO WAKING FROM THE TRANCE

Sometimes people can take an extended amount of time, 10-15 minutes, to come out of the trance. This can be natural or mean the person is really enjoying the trance.

Use your normal or more authoritative voice and say their name when talking to them.

I always tell my client 5- 15 minutes before the end of the session that they have _?_ minutes left.

EXTREME MUSCLE TENSION AND QUICK & INTENSE BREATHING

This usually means the person has remembered an old (mostly a negative) memory or experience.

- *Ask the person what they are experiencing.*
- *Listen to the tone of voice that is used.*
- *Make sure you use a more authoritative tone and ask if they want to go somewhere safe.*
- *If it is too traumatic, you might need to end the session, change it to another type of session, or refer them to a psychologist or psychiatrist.*

ANSWERS

There are a few ways to have a person answer you:

- Have the person nod the head up and down for 'yes' and side to side for 'no.'
- Have the person move their pointer finger up and down for 'yes' and side to side for 'no.'
- **Or** have the person move their left pointer finger for 'yes' and right pointer finger for 'no.'
- Have the person talk to you.

Pre-Test

Arm Levitation

Many Hypnotherapists well use this technique to determine trance ability and whether the person likes to go deeper into a trance or lighter into a trance. There are a few variations to this technique.

Procedure:

- Tell and show the person the outcome of their arm. Ask which arm would be easy to be lifted in the air. Then slowly lift their arm off their leg (if their arms are on a chair, ask them to place them on their lap) and into the air.
- Ask the person to pretend to <u>go into a trance</u> and experience all the sensations that they would experience to feel if they were in a <u>trance</u>. Lift their arm as if it were happening.
- Relax the person (see relaxation technique)
- Tell the person: (change voice tone)
  o Notice how you are sitting in your chair.
  o Notice how you feel
  o Also, notice how your arms feel.
- *Pause... (Wait a moment for them to think about what is happening)*

- o A helium balloon is lightly tied to your left wrist and will raise the arm slightly.
- o Each time a helium balloon is tied to your wrist, the arm raises slightly. You will go deeper into relaxation.
- o You will probably notice a difference to your left wrist once more helium balloons are tied onto your left wrist.
- *Pause...*

  - o Two more helium balloons are tied to your left wrist.
- *Pause...*

  - o One more helium balloon is tied to your left wrist.
  - o You will start to notice a slight difference in your left wrist.
  - o It might be lifting slightly.
  - o That's right
- *Pause...*

  - o Placed onto your right wrist is a bag. The handles are resting on your wrist, and the bag hangs towards the floor.
  - o One big rock about the size of your hand is placed into the bag on your right wrist.
  - o You may notice a difference right away from the weight and heaviness of the rock.
  - o Three more large rocks are placed into the bag hanging on your right wrist.
  - o If you like, you may re-adjust your body to handle the weight of the rocks in the bag.
- *Pause...*

  - o Two more helium balloons are tied to your left wrist.

- o Your left wrist feels much lighter, and it seems to lift off your leg into the air.
- o One more helium balloon is tied to your wrist.
- o Your wrist rises higher, hovering lightly.
- o That's right

- *Pause...*

  - o Two more big rocks are added to the bag on your right wrist.
  - o It is very heavy now.
  - o If you need to adjust your body to hold the weight.
  - o It takes some effort to keep your arm up... holding the bag off the floor.
- *Pause...*

  - o Notice the feelings in both arms and wrists.
  - o Which arm do you feel the most or moved the most?
- *Pause...*

  - o Notice where both arms are now located from the original location.
- *Bring the person out of the trance*

Ask the person to take a breath, let go of the bag, and release all balloons. Give your body a slight shake and return to normal, fully alert.

Ask their opinion of the experience.

Michael's

Ask the person the following questions about the experience by asking them to answer the questions by nodding their head yes (Demo the head nod and wait for their head to nod yes before asking any other question).

- "In a moment, there will be a change in your breathing. <u>Nod your head yes when you feel the change.</u>
- In a moment, there will be a sensation in your throat. <u>Nod your head yes when you feel this sensation.</u>
- With your eyes closed (ask them to close their eyes if not already closed) in a moment, there will be a sensation in your eyes. <u>Nod your head yes when you feel this sensation.</u>
- In a moment, you will notice a sensation in your hand (lightly stroke the hand attached to the arm you moved previously), which means your hand is starting to lift."

Begin saying the phrase in a higher tone of voice.

- "<u>Lifting and raising, lifting and raising, lifting and raising.</u>"

At any time the person's body makes any movement to indicate confirmation of the hand lifting, saying:

- "<u>That's right.</u>"
- "Your hand has a message for your face, and your face wants that message. As your hand lifts to your face, it will gently touch your face. Your face wants these wonderful insights and messages.

- Your face and hand are attached together with a string.
- One end of the string is attached to your hand, and the other to your face.
- The string is pulled in the center, bringing your hand and face together. Once they touch, you will have your message.
- That's right.

Once the hand and face touch

- Your hand is now stuck to your face. The more you try to move it away, the more it sticks to your face.
- Your hand is now free from your face, and all the string and bag are removed.
- I will count to three, and you will be fully alert and feeling wonderful with your new message.
- One
- Two
- Three, wide awake. Take a deep breath and wiggle your toes.

Inductions

The purpose of induction is for the conscious mind to have something to do while the subconscious is accessible. As soon as a person gets out of their head and focuses on their body, the mind goes into a trance state. You want the person to concentrate on something else. The focal point is relaxation.

To bring a person into a trance will take a bit of time, anywhere from five to twenty minutes. You might have to do more than one induction type to relax a person.

Progressive Relaxation is intended to deliberately relax and tense the body, usually just relaxing each part of the body from toes to head, front, and back. Describing soothing surroundings such as the forest or ocean or experiences like swimming, scuba diving, and walking will relax many people.

Breath Method

Having the person concentrate on their breathing while you say relaxing statements or sentences will bring a person into a trance.

- Deep breath, slowly.
- Notice your breathing going in and out.
- Count how long it takes to breathe in
- Hold for the same count
- Out for the same count
- Continue breathing slowly

Do count method or Imagery to finish induction.

Spot Method

- Have the person stare at a spot above eye level.
- Deep breath
- Notice how tired your eyes are getting
- Tell yourself, "My eyes are getting tired, sleepy, and heavy. They only want to close.

Do count method or Imagery to finish induction.

Imagery Method (safe place)

- Make yourself really comfortable.
- Close your eyes.
- Breathe deeply
- Go to your safe place. This safe place is only for you. Only you can go there. No one is allowed to enter your safe space without your permission.
- Make yourself very comfortable.
- *If you want to ask your client about their safe space, ask them now.*
- Imagine all the smells, colors, sounds, sights, noises, feelings, thoughts, and tastes you have in your safe place.
- This safe place is your haven. Every time you go here, you will relax, rejuvenate and recharge.

Go into your hypnosis session from here.

Internalization

- Notice your breath.
- Do not change it; simply be aware of your breathing.
- Notice any sensations that you are feeling, seeing, hearing, or thinking.
- Observe them.
- Begin to pay attention to even more subtle sensations.
- Notice how your lungs move.
- Your mind may feel like drifting
- Let go and relax

Go into your hypnosis session from here

If using it for going to sleep, *say, "Wake up in your usual manner."*

Count Method

Every number should coincide with the person's breathing

- Imagine you are about to go up (*or* down) 10 (20, 50, 100) steps of a spiral stairway, and with every step, you feel sleeper and sleeper (*or* deeper and deeper relaxed *or* lighter and lighter).
- Go ahead and take your first step, one...
- Two...three...four... you are feeling (sleeper / more relaxed / lighter) five... (all the way to ?...).
- Ten (or the end of the counting), you are deeply asleep / extremely relaxed / light as a feather.

Go into your hypnosis session from here.

Fascination

This is where a person focuses on a spot, spiral disc, swinging watch (pendulum), or any other object. As the person focuses on the object, do another induction method.

Fractionation Method

This method uses a rhythm that has a relaxing and deepening effect on the person.

You can use this as an induction or a deepening technique.

1. A fractionation counting technique would be 1-5 and then 5-0
   - "I am going to count from 1-5 and 5-0. When I say 0, you will be completely and very deeply relaxed. (pace the person's breath)
   - One, (on out-breath)
   - Two...
   - Three...
   - Four, and deeper
   - Five...
   - Four...
   - Three...
   - Two...
   - One (pause)
   - Completely and very deeply relaxed...Zero
2. A fractionation visual technique would be walking over green grassy hills or watching waves.

This technique involves a sensation of up-and-down motion

   - "I would like you to imagine lying or sitting on a beach.
   - You are watching the waves wash up on shore and onto the sand.
   - Noticing the wave rise and then fall as it hits the shoreline.
   - And the next wave behind that.

- As each wave rises to shore, you will go deeper and deeper into relaxation.
- As each wave touches the sand, you will go deeper and deeper into trance.
- After about ten (20, 30...) waves touching the shore, the waves will disappear, and you will be deeply relaxed and comfortable".

3. A fractionation kinesthetic technique would be to have the person focus on the sound of the waves hitting the beach or have a person go into sleep and then out and then back in. (Vogt's)
   - "I am now going to awaken you by counting to five.
   - After I have done that...
   - And even though your eyes are open...
   - You will begin to feel very, very drowsy and sleepy again.
   - You will find it harder and harder to keep your eyes open and stay awake.
   - Your eyes will feel very, very heavy.
   - The eyelids will feel heavier.
   - And will begin to blink.
   - You will not be able to stop them from blinking.
   - And as they blink, you will find it more and more difficult to keep them open.
   - They will want to close.
   - You will not be able to stop them from closing.
   - Every moment as I go on talking...
   - You will feel drowsier and drowsier...
   - Sleepier and sleepier.
   - Your eyes will close, and you will fall into a deep sleep.
   - You will be in a much deeper sleep than you are now.
   - I am going to count slowly up to five.

- As I do so, you will open your eyes and wake up.
- But you will feel very, very drowsy...
- Very, very tired.
- So tired that you will not be able to keep them open for very long.
- They will start to blink.
- You will be unable to stop them from blinking.
- And as they do so, your eyes will feel very tired.
- That they will close.
- And you will fall into a much, much deeper sleep.
- *Count to the number five*
- You see, your eyes are feeling heavier and heavier.
- You are feeling very, very drowsy and sleepy.
- Your eyes are closing.
- And you are falling into a deeper, deeper sleep.
- Go to sleep.
- You see, your eyes have closed on their own.
- Sleep very, very deeply.
- Very, very deeply".

Confusion Method

It is used to confuse the person to the extreme and give them a logical option. The confusion method consists of ambiguous statements or plays on words. Any use of crazy play on words to create a 'HUH,' where you can present a desirable option. An example from Bennett/Stellar is, *Take the words right, write, rite, and Wright. As you right about the Wright brothers, you realize you have violated the rights of those whose right this is by righting with your right hand instead of your left.* After saying this statement, you pause and then add ...*and that makes you feel really silly!*

This method consists of sets of six statements.

- The first set contains five (5) accurate/logical descriptions of the present experience and one (1) abstract / illogical description. (you will feel more and more relaxed with every breath you take...the more relaxed you get, the safer you feel...weirdly enough, these bring back memories of John Smith's blue healer).
- The Second consists of four (4) accurate/logical descriptions of the present experience and two (2) abstract/illogical descriptions.
- The third consists of three (3) accurate/logical descriptions of the present experience and three (3) abstract / illogical descriptions.
- The forth consists of two (2) accurate/logical descriptions of the present experience and four (4) abstract / illogical descriptions.
- The Fifth consists of one (1) accurate/logical description of the present experience and five (5) abstract / illogical descriptions.
- The last one consists of all (6) abstract / illogical descriptions.

Quick Method

Usually used by stage hypnotists since the audience's attention span is not long. When you have the time, use the other methods of trance.

Handshake method

Walk up to the person and say

- "I am going to shake your hand three times. The first time your eyes will get tired... let them.
- The second time they will want to close...Let them.
- The third time they will lock, and you will not be able to open them...
- I want that to happen and watch that happen.
- Start to shake the person's hand

- Now, one...two...
- Now close your eyes...
- Now three...and they are locked
- And you will find they just will not work no matter how hard you try.
- The harder you try, the less they will work.
- Test them.
- And you will find that they won't work at all".

Coin Method

The person extends their arm about even with their shoulder, palm facing up. Place a coin (quarter or larger) on the ulnar edge of the hand (pinky side).

Saying:

- "Please fix your eyes as long as they are open upon the coin.
- I will start counting.
- With each count, the hand will slowly turn over and inward until soon, the coin falls off.
- When the coin falls, your eyes will close as if they are not already shut.
- And you will become completely relaxed.
- The arm will fall as if it were dead weight.
- The other muscles of the body will relax completely".
- *Make sure the person does not fall!*

Deepening Techniques

1. **Counting** – "I am going to count from 10-1. The closer I get to one, the deeper you can go into a trance".
2. **Breath** – "With every breath you take, the deeper you will go into a trance."
3. **Sound** – "With the sound of the waves hitting the shore, you will go deeper and deeper into a trance." (Seashore music, Tibetan bells, or any sound that the subject enjoys).
4. **Imagery** – "With every step you take down the stairs you will go deeper into a trance." (Walking on a beach, floating on a cloud, etc.)
5. **Double Induction** - After the first induction, have the person open their eyes and then tell them that they will go even deeper into a trance when they close their eyes again.

Studies have shown that the vibrations from rhythmic sounds profoundly affect brain activity. In shamanic traditions, drums were used-in periodic rhythm to transport the shaman into other realms of reality. The vibrations from this constant rhythm affected the brain specifically, allowing the shaman to journey out of their body.

Re-Inducing Hypnosis

Your person may want to have a word, symbol, or gesture to reinstate hypnosis on their next visit. Whatever the person would like to imagine will work. You never will want the association activated while they drive, so pick something safe.

Having the person remember the last session brings many persons back to the trance state.

I like to use their safe place.

Say all of this to the person:

"I am going to count from one to three; at the count of three, you will be relaxed and into a trance.

- One: you are noticing your breathing going in and out slowly.
- Two: your whole body relaxes.
- Three: you are deeply relaxed."

Or

"I am going to count from one to three, and at the count of three, I will say 'sleep' and snap my fingers. That will signal you to shut your eyes and go deep into a trance.

- One
- Two
- Three: "sleep" (snap fingers)

Or

Go to 'Safe Place.'

Hypnotherapy Session

- Interview the Person
- Pre-Frame
- Anchor
- The purpose for the Session/Procedure
- Posthypnotic Suggestion
- Terminate

Interview the Person

What is the reason for the session?

If the person has never been hypnotized before, you may want to practice a rehearsed trance (Pre-test) that brings the person in and out of the trance.

Pre-Frame

Explain what you will do and what might be expected.

This is where you would tell the person what to expect before entering a trance. Your voice will change on specific <u>words</u> or <u>sentences</u>. You want to emphasize these to the person, subtle subconscious mind recognition.

"I will explain a few things before you <u>go into a trance</u>. I will guide you <u>to relax your body</u>. You can keep your eyes open <u>or closed</u> during the session. It will not influence the session one way or the other, whatever makes you comfortable. And if you ever want out of what we are doing in the session at any time, you can open your eyes or go back <u>to your safe place</u>. From <u>your safe place,</u> we will do what you have asked for your session.

I am not always sure what will come up since it is your session, but I will tell you what we will be doing ahead of time. In a trance you will be going into a <u>deep hypnotic trance.</u> Many people find this like <u>mediation</u>.

Okay, take a deep breath and make yourself very comfortable".

Continue to the 'Anchor.'

Anchor

Anchor problem/issue to the conscious mind and solution to the subconscious mind.

Goal = now to the conscious mind and outcome to the subconscious mind.

This is where the mind tells the difference between the problem and the desired outcome.

You can do this by saying:

- "I am talking to the conscious mind only now (say what the problem is). Listen very closely to every word". Example: Conscious mind, you have told me you want to lose weight. You do not feel good about how you look... etc.
- If this is true, nod your head (or whichever way you have set up for the person to answer).
- "I am now talking to the subconscious mind only (say what the outcome will be).
- Example: Subconscious mind, you have told me you want to be ten pounds lighter. Be more toned and have extra energy... etc.
- If this is true, nod your head.
- Great, we are ready to move on.

Continue to the 'Induction.'

Induction

Choose an induction to bring the person into a trance. You may use more than one if you think it is needed.

Continue to the 'Purpose for the session.'

Purpose For the Session/Procedure

This is where you do the counseling part of the session. Reframe/change old belief system to new belief system.

Problem:

Outcome:

Intention:

Highest Intention:

Common Abilities:

The transformation theme:

Posthypnotic suggestion

Direct - statement

Indirect – subtle or presupposed outcome.

You will use your version or a scripted version for the session.

Many practitioners write a script of their own and like to be spontaneous and make it up as they go. Whatever works for you, if you are more comfortable in the beginning to follow a prewritten script, yours or someone else's is okay.

Depending on what outcome you are trying for will determine what script you use.

The person can tell you the issue, and under hypnosis, they can tell you the best way to fix it.

Continue to the 'Post Hypnotic Suggestion.'

Post-Hypnotic Suggestion

This is any suggestion you gave to a person in the hypnotic state to have a specific effect even after the session.

- "Every time you say 'good morning,' you will feel happy.
- "From now on, whenever I say the word 'NOW,' you will immediately go into a deep, relaxed state."
- "From now on, whenever you take a deep breath, you will completely relax".

- Anytime I say the word 'SLEEP NOW', you will go into a deep sleep".
- "When you awaken from this session you will feel revived and refreshed".
- "You have the power to do your best and achieve your dreams. Your future is full of great opportunities".

Continue to the 'Termination of the Session.'

Terminate

As long as the person is not going to sleep for the night and there is no suggestion to undo (For example, in Arm levitation, one arm is heavy, and one is light). You would bring the person back to normal or better than normal.

Termination: Say all of this to the person:

"Now I am going to count from five to one, and at the count of one, I will say, "wide awake.' You will be fully awake, calm, rested, refreshed, and relaxed."

"All right,

- Five: slowly, calmly, and easily you are returning to your full awareness.
- Four: all your muscles and nerves are loose and relaxed.
- Three: from head to toe, you feel perfect in every way. Physically, emotionally, mentally, and spiritually.
- Two: you can wiggle your toes and fingers.

- One: wide awake, opening your eye, stretching, feeling wonderful."

Or

- Take a deep breath.
- Wiggle your toes.
- And open your eyes.
- Coming back to the present moment.
- Feeling great.

You can also return to your regular voice.

Give the person a moment and then ask the person how they feel and to tell you about the session.

I sometimes ask, what was the best thing they learned through the session? Or what they received out of the session?

Not that this is normal, but if the person feels dizzy or not quite awake, you can re-hypnotize her and then suggest feeling great and awake; having a drink of water or using the bathroom works also. Just ensure they are better than when they came in to see you, and she is safe to drive home.

Hypnotherapy Procedures

You can use one or more of these ideas in the 'Purpose for the session' section.

Safe Place

I have clients create a safe place before I do ANY counseling Hypnotherapy.

Once the person is in a trance, have them imagine a safe place. It can be indoors or out, anywhere in the world, or the universe, for that matter. Anywhere they feel absolutely safe.

I say, "Imagine a safe place that only you are allowed to be in... Imagine 360° around you... beneath you, on top, and all around you... This is a sacred space that only you can be in... no one else can enter your space... it is forbidden. This is your space... they have their own space...

Now describe it to me...

- What it looks like,
- (_____their answer)
- Are there any sounds,
- (_____their answer)
- Are there any Smells,
- (_____their answer)

- (if outside) Can you feel the wind or temperature?
- (_____their answer)
- Are they sitting or standing, or lying down?
- (_____their answer)

Then I say, "Make yourself comfortable... relax and enjoy... this space is for you to come to any time you need to rejuvenate...relax and enjoy...

This is the place I want you to come to any time during the session... you can come here if you need a break from the session... or get scared...

And this will be the place that sometimes I will ask you to go to... sometimes when I need to think of better questions or if I need to write things down from what you said, I will ask you to go to your safe place...

Do you understand? (_____their answer)

From here in the session, I move on to one of the other procedures.

Story Mode

I use this procedure a lot. It is one of my favorites.

Once the person is in a trance and you have done the safe place... have the person imagine they are the main actor/actress in a movie **and** the script is being written.

Have the person think of their issue...

I say, "Imagine that you are at a train station... this is a very special train. It will go backward in time... when you step off this train, it will be at the perfect time in history that corresponds to your issue...

Go ahead and buy your train ticket...
Now go to your train and hop on...
Find a seat... You can choose to be facing in the direction the train will be heading or sit on the opposite side...
If you brought luggage, store it now...
The conductor comes and checks everyone's ticket and punches a hole in the corner to show you have used your ticket...
The conductor calls out, "All aboard"...
And the train's engine starts up...
The train starts to move slowly backward in time...
You are comfortable on the train and can look out the window, read, chat with others, or do anything you would normally like to do...
The train picks up speed...
...
In a moment, the train will start to slow down...
This is your stop...
The train slows down and comes to a stop at the new station...
As you get your things and get ready to leave the train...

Please step to the side once you are outside of the train and allow others to go past you...
Go ahead and get off the train, stepping to the side...

I would like you to look at your feet... What are you wearing?
(_____their answer), *write it down on paper.*

What clothes are you wearing?
(_____their answer), *write it down on paper.*

Are you male or female? If you need to, walk over to a window, water puddle, mirror, or reflective surface.
(_____their answer), *write it down on paper.*

What age are you, or your approximate age?
(_____their answer), *write it down on paper.*

What year or era is it? If you need to walk over to a paper stand and look at the date.
(_____their answer), *write it down on paper.*

What season is it?
(_____their answer), *write it down on paper.*

Is this a town/city/village?
(_____their answer), *write it down on paper.*

Do you live in town or out of town?
(_____their answer), *write it down on paper.*

Teleport, walk, drive, take a taxi, horse-drawn carriage, anything, and quickly go to where you live. Please tell me when you are there.

What does their home look like?
(_____their answer), *write it down on paper.*

Are they married?
(_____their answer), *write it down on paper.*

If so, what kind of personality do they have?
(_____their answer), *write it down on paper.*

Do they have any children? How many?
(_____their answer), *write it down on paper.*

What do you do for work?
(_____their answer), *write it down on paper.*

Any pets?
(_____their answer), *write it down on paper.*

How do you die in this movie? How?
(_____their answer), *write it down on paper.*

What was the importance of this script/life?
(_____their answer), *write it down on paper.*

What was the purpose of this main character's life?
(_____their answer), *write it down on paper.*

What lesson did you learn in this life?
(_____their answer), *write it down on paper.*

Anything else of importance that you need to tell me?
(_____their answer), *write it down on paper.*

Once the person is finished telling you the story, have the person notice if there is any resemblance to their life.
(_____their answer), *write it down on paper.*

And what can they learn from the story?
(_____their answer), *write it down on paper.*

Terminate the session or bring the person to their safe place and proceed to ask more questions, talk to the person, or make notes.

Story mode allows the person's subconscious mind to create a story that can give symbolism or what is happening in their life today.

Sometimes having the person do the story mode procedure is all they need, but sometimes they need to move the issue out of their body.

- From here, I may go on and bring them back onto the train and do another story,
- Or, from their safe place, I might do
  - 'Different Viewpoint,'
  - Age,
  - Timeline,
  - Genealogy,
  - Kinesthetic Point Healing,
- Sometimes I may switch and bring them out of their trance and have them do a counseling technique, as in the Emotional Clearing Technique,
- Or, depending on the time left, I may end today's session and have them come in for another session,
- Or they may be finished and not need another session. I usually muscle test to see if we are finished.

Different Viewpoint

Once the person is in a trance and you have done the safe place... have the person tell you about their situation.

Write down anything that seems important.

Look at the situation from a different viewpoint. (Always re-ask the person to re-tell the situation from the other viewpoint)
- Have the person tell you what perspective they are looking from. Once they have that determined, have them choose a different viewpoint. E.g., looking down/bird's eye view, straight ahead, from the side.
- Or have them look at a T.V. screen, and they have control of the T.V. program with remote control.

Example

- From the position that you are in while you are telling me your situation, I would now like you to imagine that you are a bird looking down on yourself. What changes, differences, or discrepancies do you notice?
- From the position behind you, what now do you notice?
- From a child's point of view, what do you notice now?
- From an older person's point of view, what do you notice now?
- *You make a point of view to notice.*

Age

Your unconscious mind knows how to organize your memories. You know that what you remember is from the past week, month, year, 10 years ago, or intended for future plans that will be happening in a week or so.

Some people recall a childhood memory and attaches the memory from a certain age to the school or teacher they had or a house or city they lived in.

To find out how a person stores their memories in a timeline, ask them, "If you knew what direction your past is, what direction would you point?" or "If you knew what direction your future is, what direction would you point?"

5-10% of the people who answer <u>will not</u> know in which direction. If this happens, ask them, "Could you recall a happy memory from the age of, let us say, 14..., 20... or 30? Now notice these memories and if it implies a line. And now notice something that is going to happen in a week from now, two weeks from now? Do these memories imply a line?

Releasing a memory that is a past issue will be beneficial. It will put **the** order of importance on the issue. It may also show whose issue it is (not all issues are the persons. Some people take on their mother or father's issues).

Once the person is in a trance and you have done the safe place... have the person tell you about their situation. What age are they?

Write down anything that seems important.

- Have them be their age today and go back to their younger self and protect them, tell them they love them, tell them it will be okay because _____.

Example

- I want you to imagine that you are the age you are today. Now imagine today you go back to a younger version of you. What would you say to the younger you?
- What would you do differently?
- What could you change?
- What emotions would you change?
- Hug yourself,
- Gift your younger self something that could shift the energy to a positive,
- *? you make up something.*

Ancestry

To find out in what generation an issue originates.

Example #1
Many years ago, while attending an NLP course in the USA, the instructor did a timeline demo on me. I had to think of a situation I wanted to improve my life. So, I decided I wanted to know why the women on my Mom's side were the way they were, controlling and a bit angry.

The instructor had me imagine that I was hovering above my head and then asked me how many generations I needed to go back to find the origin of the women with this trait. I had to go back five generations (imagine going backward in time). Mine was one, my Mom was two, my grandmother was three, my great-grandmother was four, and then her mother was five generations. I was to glance down and see what was happening. The first thought was disaster and death. All I could see were dead people everywhere. All I knew about this five generations ago grandmother was that she lived in Czechoslovakia.

Then the instructor had me go back one more generation to her mother (six generations back) and look at what was happening in her life. I noticed a big difference. Her life was peaceful and happy, and easy-going, nothing like the fifth-generation grandmother's life. This grandma's life was peaceful and happy, whereas her daughter's was disastrous, painful, and bitter.

So, the instructor had me choose what type of life I wanted to follow. I decided to select the sixth-generation grandmother's personality instead.

I took from this experience that to understand something. It is better to have many perspectives before choosing my destiny. I also found it amazing how one person can affect so many others. Their emotions seemed to be passed down through the generations.

The **secret** to releasing a memory is to go before the negative memory begins and notice a positive or neutral feeling about that memory. The different perspectives will shift your thought to a new way of thinking.

Example #2
A little bit different, but it worked just as well.
It was a time in my life when I was new in my school and felt like I was being judged and felt like I could not win, that there were too many people that I felt were attacking me (five to be exact).

I did a meditation and, in it, asked God what I do about this. God answered to have me float above my house, city, and country, right up into space, and look back on the world. To take note of these five people and envision them as lights. I say five red lights.

Next, I was told to note all the students that wanted me to be a school, now in the future. I started to notice all these little white lights lighting up worldwide *(from space, the earth was turning).* When I came out of the meditation, it gave me a wonderful feeling and a purpose not to give up.

And over the years, I have developed into an accredited college and have many graduated students worldwide. Mostly due to this new vision!

Kinesthetic Point Healing

This is used to connect the neurons connected with the sensation of touch and the re-programming of an issue/memory using the emotional state as the trigger.

Kinesthetic Point Healing Procedure
Have the person remember a good memory.

- Touch (slowly and lightly, tap) a spot on the person (*that they have permitted you to touch*) while they are thinking of a beautiful or enjoyable thought.
- Have them remember the memory again but amp up the excellent memory by making it even 10x better.
- Now 20x better while still tapping.
- Release your finger (Take your finger off of the person)

Have the person now think of the negative issue that they want to clear or replace

- Choose another spot (2nd spot on the person's body); lightly tapping makes the person think of the negative emotion.
- Do the negative a few times
- Release your finger (Take your finger off of the person)

Now both together

- 1st -Touch and <u>hold</u> the negative spot
- Now at the same time, touch the excellent memory spot and <u>hold both</u>
  - **(This must always be in this order, or you will create a good memory to become bad!)**
- *You should be touching both spots now*
- *Hold for about the count of 30 seconds*

- Release both places at the same time
- Do both again
    - Touch and <u>hold</u> the negative spot
    - Now touch the good memory spot and <u>hold</u> at the same time
    - *You should be touching both places for the count of 30 seconds*
- Repeat the hold of both spots 3x in total (negative spot first, then good spot)

Now touch the negative spot <u>only</u> and ask what is happening now. The emotion should be gone or dissipated.

If not, redo the whole session and up the excellent memory or choose a better good memory. You can have them see it, hear, feel, taste, and smell it to the best of their ability by 100x or 1000x

- Repeat the procedure if need be.

I have found over time that if the person was in a drunken or altered state (drugs) at the time of the memory, this will probably not work.

Phobias

The main objective is to distort the memory. There are many ways to do this.

Example one:
- Have the person remember the negative memory/phobia
- Have them imagine that they are now jumping on the memory like a trampoline
- You can even have them safely jump through the trampoline making a hole in it.
- Next, have them imagine the trampoline turns into paper, and they have funky scissors that can cut up the paper into shapes or designs.
- Imagine all the pieces being scooped up and packed into a ball that can fit into the size of a basketball, and you start to bounce it.
- The hoop is connected to a cosmic vacuum cleaner. As you make a perfect shot into the basket, the negative memory is sucked up by the vacuum forever.

Another example: For a spider phobia
- Imagine the spider
- Imagine the spider having bright pink lipstick put on its lips
- And long eyelashes
- Maybe a fluffy ballet tutu
- And having fussy kitten feet
- And you can take a feather and tickle it, and it dances like a ballet dancer
- Now make the spider either really, really large, like where it cannot even step on earth, or so small that

it is tinier than a fruit fly or sand fly, smaller than the tip of a needle.

- And the spider is so dissatisfied with how you preserve it; it leaves your presence forever.

You can take any phobia and distort the realism of it. You can make up any combination.

Or maybe you can have the person imagine that they are the spider and experience life as a spider through the spider's perspective. How it feels, thinks, eats, sees, hears, what it fears, and how that feels.

Ericksonian Style Hypnotherapy

Milton H. Erickson, M.D. was performing Hypnotherapy sessions even from his wheelchair. Milton believed that each person was unique. He was color-blind, tone-deaf, dyslexic, and became paralyzed from polio. He thought no two people were alike, and you could not cookie-cut a session. You would need to consider the person's; beliefs, behavior, motivations, symptoms, etc., and create a unique session for that person.

Every person will have a different experience while in a trance, and it is not the hypnotist but the person with control. You aim to stimulate the person's attention to their memories, body sensations, thoughts, emotions, feelings, ideas, past learning, and experiences.

When you, as the practitioner, suggest an idea, it can only happen if the person believes it is true. Your goal is to use the person's knowledge of the issue and use that in the session. Take the issue and play with it. Find out if the person has thought of it differently or challenged it. You would use the person's issue to find out the skill or resource they already have because of it and use it as a transformational strategy and/or reorganize the relevant memories and beliefs.

The Ericksonian style of hypnosis focuses on the goal, not the past issue. Using the positive and not dwelling on the negative (a solution is a primary aspect). The conscious mind works linearly, and the unconscious mind works holistically. The unconscious mind looks after the body and will protect itself even if the conscious mind wants something.

An example would be someone who wants to stop smoking and has tried before. The mind knows what it had to go through the first time; pain, discomfort, etc., and decides it is too much and does not want to create that situation again. Hence, the subconscious mind decides it would be better for the whole body, mind, and spirit if it does not go through that turmoil again, so the person does not stop smoking. Using hypnosis, you would have to discover any subconscious issues as to why the mind would not want to quit smoking (good or bad) and use that information for the person to digest and decide what next step to choose to take. It must be the person's decision for a successful change.

INTEGRITY

This may be an essential aspect of your being successful. D.O. you have the person's best wishes in mind, or is your ego involved? Trust and honesty... you need to be in line with your person. Know what your intentions are.
Support the person's journey for change.
Set aside your biased opinions.
Do not put your ideas or personal beliefs onto the person.

TRADITIONAL VS. ERICKSONIAN
STYLE OF HYPNOSIS

Traditional Method of Hypnosis from 1964

Pre-induction

Establish Report

Diagnosis Problem

Identify and dispel myths

Establish 'diagnoses' through suggestibility tests.

Induction

Whichever method you want to start with, e.g., relaxation

Deepening

Direct suggestion

Using a scale

Fractionation

Provide a test for any hypnotic phenomenon

Therapy

Positive Suggestion

Negative Suggestion

Termination

Return control to the subject

Re-establish conscious support

Re-establish conscious set

Ratify the trance (time)

ERICKSONIAN HYPNOSIS

Guide attention

Build responsiveness

Guide association

Utilize confusion to disrupt the conscious set

Promote disassociation

1. Pattern perceptional change
2. Establish regression
3. Access the motivation
4. Ratify the responses as hypnotic
5. Define the situation as hypnosis

***Watch any YouTube videos of **Milton H. Erickson's live hypnosis session.**

ERICKSONIAN HYPNOTIC STYLE
(PLASTICITY OF PERCEPTION)

1. Sensory
   a. Hallucinations
   b. Anesthesia
   c. Analgesic
   d. Catalepsy
2. Autonomic behavior/disassociation
   a. Ideomotor behavior
   b. Ideosensory behavior
   c. Automatic behavior
   d. Posthypnotic suggestion
3. Time reference
   a. Time distortion
4. Memory functions
   a. Amnesia
   b. Hyper amnesia
   c. Age regression

A great book to read is "My Voice Will Go With You, the teaching tales of Milton H. Erickson," by Sidney Rosen ISBN: 780393301359

Scripts

Quit Smoking

Hypnosis session for Stop Smoking *(negative)*

Induce the trance state...*(your choice of induction)*

First, you know we have already completely uncovered the underlying cause of your compulsive smoking habit... You no longer feel the compulsion to smoke at all... We are now only dealing with a habit pattern — the hollow shell of your original problem...

Habits can be broken as quickly as they are created... One of the ways to do that is to make you aware of your smoking... From the very moment you reach for a cigarette, you will be extremely conscious of what you are doing... If you light it and start to smoke, you will be unusually aware of every moment of the time you are involved in smoking that cigarette... You have continued to smoke mainly because you are doing it <u>un</u>consciously... you have not really been aware of what you were doing... But you are now...

Each time you reach for a cigarette, your attention will be drawn to that cigarette and focus uncomfortably upon it...

When you are aware of what you're doing, you are no longer in the <u>un</u>conscious habit... You already do not need to continue smoking; you know that... So this will be easy and effortless... There will be none of the struggles and fight with willpower you may have experienced in the past... no guilt of how long you had smoked for as you quit forever... The awareness may make you annoyed with smoking, disgusted, and bored by it... You may even want to put the cigarette out when you are only half-finished...

The cigarette will not taste as good as it used to... You simply will not wish to continue... You have already made up your mind... You have found the reason you smoke, and you have already made up your mind... a final decision to stop smoking altogether... You have already made up your mind to stop smoking altogether...You have already made up your mind that you will stop now, not tomorrow, not the next day, but you will stop this very moment. ..You have made a final decision to stop smoking forever...

You want to stop smoking as of this very minute... You know why you want to quit... Think about that reason...

Form it clearly in your mind... Think about the problems smoking causes... You have no need to smoke anymore... you are giving it up for good... You're giving up coughing... you're giving up pain... you're giving up the expense... you're giving up the inconvenience...you're giving up all the things you don't want, including smoking... You are giving up the things you don't want to

get the things you want... relaxation, rest, a feeling of security, health, and happiness...
You will forget about cigarettes altogether... You do not have to buy them ever again... because you have no need to smoke them... Consequently, your purchase of cigarettes will immediately cease... And should you perhaps accept a cigarette without realizing it, you will immediately be aware of it and will be overcome with an uncontrollable compulsion to break it in two as soon as it enters your hand...

Whenever you touch the cigarette, you will instantly break it in two... It will remind you of all the bad things you are giving up and all the good things in store for you... You realize how much greater the proportion of good you receive is than the portion of bad you are giving up... It will seem small to you to give up smoking, considering the tremendous benefits you will receive for giving it up... It is easy to give up things you do not like... And from today, you do not want to smoke...

You will begin to feel proud of yourself, very proud... You will find it easier to conquer other habits... It makes it easier for you to conquer life in general... It fills your ego, making you self-confident, self-assured, and self-reliant...

You will keep a record at the beginning of your progress... Every single day, you will remind yourself how successful you have been as an abstainer... How many days and weeks and months have you been an abstainer and how wonderful it has made you feel... You will continue to keep this record, and it will encourage you and fortify you as a reliable record of your success... And soon, you will no longer feel the need to keep such a record because you will know that you are an abstainer permanently... That this record will go on unblemished for the rest of your life...

You already know that no habit is stronger than the power of your mind, which created it in the first place. ..It is now you versus tobacco... You will easily win, for you are stronger... You have patience, great patience now, perseverance, great perseverance, calm, and relaxed determination... Nothing can shake it... You will go on patiently day today. Every day will be a success... You will become accustomed to success... And soon that feeling of success will be far more critical to you than any habit could possibly be...

Take a deep breath and wiggle your toes and fingers, returning to this moment, feeling empowered and in control of your success...

Quit Smoking Script #2

Induce a trance state...

You pay attention only to the sound of my voice... Sink further and further down, deeper and deeper... Sleep deeply... Sleep... Deeper and deeper... As you listen to the sound of my voice, your mind concentrates on it... It is easy for your mind to focus, concentrating to a pinpoint... You find you will be able to concentrate on your work and your play and concentrate at all times... It makes you feel good and feel relaxed... For when your mind is concentrating on other things, there is no room for smoking to even get into it... When you become fatigued or tired, you can lie down for a couple of minutes, go into a state of self-hypnosis, and relax completely... Because concentrating on the mind does not make it tired... The mind becomes fatigued out of confusion, not concentration...

Smoking has been a form of self-punishment, a way of feeding yourself poison that you neither like nor need... You only need this when you make yourself tired and tell yourself that you are consciously on your way to death. That is not true... Tiredness is merely a sign that you need to rejuvenate yourself, which can be done easily with self-hypnosis... Smoking is more than a crutch - a hindrance, a block in your path... We are removing that block... We are wiping it out entirely so you can go on to success as if it had been erased... The wall is no longer there... You walk straight ahead and wipe out smoking completely so it has no place in your life...

It is not a substitute for anything - not for death or self-punishment or anything else... It is a nonentity...It does not exist for you... It has been wiped out by your concentrating on other beneficial things... As you think of your goals, work, and play, the idea of smoking never appears... It vanishes completely... You have no use for it... It is a good substitute for nothing... Indeed, you are surprised and amazed at how easy it is for you to concentrate your mind on everything you want to... Your goals...your aspirations...your desires...your needs...your work and relaxation...

Smoking is gone from your thoughts... And with it is gone all the poison, all the negative suggestions, all the self-punishment and degradation, and all the problems... A cycle for good has been established...The more you hear these words, the more they will take effect on you, for even as you listen to them in the deepest part of your subconscious mind, these suggestions take effect, complete and thorough effect in every way...sealing themselves into the deepest part of your subconscious mind, and becoming an integral part of each and every cell of your brain and body, making you more healthy and more satisfied in every way and feeling good all over...

Now I want you to take five very deep breaths...I want you to breathe in the very deepest, cleanest, most wonderful air into your lungs... There's one... Now let it out... Feel how wonderful that feels... There's no smoke there... Nothing to do with it... Two...take a deep breath...all the way in, all the way out... Feel the air reach the very distant recesses of every single part of your lungs... Three... as this happens, you gain a tremendous desire... breathe all the way out... tremendous desire, what wonderful clean, fresh air. Four - and the wonderful feeling it gives you as you breathe in all the way in and all the way out... And on this last breath that is coming in, you realize how much you enjoy breathing clear, pure, fresh air without smoke or irritants of any kind... It's wonderful to you... All the way in, all the way in, all the way in, further and further and further...the deepest breath you have ever taken in your life...all the way down, that develops in you a desire for deep, comfortable, wonderful breathing such as accomplished in healthy, comfortable, satisfied people like yourself... As you continue in this way, continue to breathe comfortably, feel good...concentrate your mind on those things that need concentrating on... Every day, in every way, you are getting better and better and better...

Now I'm going to give you a short period of silence during which each one of those suggestions will take complete and thorough effect upon you...sealing themselves into the deepest part of your subconscious mind and reinforcing themselves over and over again... All these suggestions and any other suggestions I have given you, are now reinforced... Again and again and again... That time begins now...

Five minutes later

...Wonderful... All these suggestions and any other suggestions I have given you are now reinforced...every time you take a breath in and out... reinforced...in and out...

Take a deep breath and wiggle your toes and fingers, returning to this moment, feeling empowered and in control...

Weight Reduction Script

Induction of your choice...or

Please relax...and make yourself comfortable...closing your eyes when you are ready...not falling asleep...listening to my voice...but very, very relaxed...

Please bring your focus to your feet...imagine that there are cosmic vacuum cleaners attached to each foot...removing any negative energy that you no longer require...breathing in...and out...relaxing more and more...bringing in good fresh energy with your breath in and releasing everything you no longer need with your breath out...relaxing...breathing in and out...

Next, concentrate on your legs, calves, and thighs...breathing in and out... releasing and relaxing... breathing in and out...now focus on your torso; chest, breasts, hips, and stomach...breathing in and out...in and out...release and relax...now concentrate on your shoulders, arms, hands and fingers...again, release and relax... breathing in and out...in and out...and lastly your neck and face; relax your mouth, ears, eyes, cheeks and even your hair...relax and release... breathing in and out...

Enjoy this wonderful feeling of total relaxation...still able to listen to what I am saying, but very deeply relaxed...now relax your mental state...you are going to count down from 100 to 97...and with each number, you will again go deeper and deeper into relaxation...100...relaxing even more...99...even more relaxed than before...98...breathing in and out...even more relaxed...and 97...total and completely relaxed...able to hear my voice but completely relaxed...

You have chosen to begin your positive approach to obtaining a slim, healthy, and attractive body, which you desire... I am going to give you some suggestions that will make this a permanent change in your living... Your mind will easily accept these suggestions, which are going to take complete and thorough effect upon the deepest part of your subconscious mind... sealing themselves in the deepest part of your subconscious mind, so they will remain there forever and become a permanent part of every cell of your brain and body...

You are going to be surprised and amazed at just how effective these suggestions are going to be... and how much they will become a part of your everyday life...giving you a brand new pattern...brand new thoughts...a brand new method of action, to make you an effective and successful person...

You will make use of this brand-new method which you may have never used before... you have begun the first positive approach for obtaining the healthy, attractive body which you desire...you have chosen hypnosis as a positive means to attain this goal...because hypnosis is a great aid in permanently changing your emotional reactions to food and eating... You realize that hypnosis is a new positive approach... a new positive approach to obtain what you desire...

You will really initiate a good positive approach toward food and eating... As you initiate this positive attitude toward food... enjoy healthy food, like healthy foods, and eat healthy foods... You will create a permanent positive change in your eating habits... From now on...you will prove to your own satisfaction that eating all that your body needs...fruit and vegetables, for the minerals and vitamins... meat, nuts, and dairy for the protein, to build healthy muscles...good fats like; flax, olive or grapeseed oil for the brain...and fiber from flaked grains to help clean the colon and bowels...these foods will entirely satisfy you...as well as drinking all the water you need...

We do not suggest that you try to kill your appetite, treating it as an enemy... instead you are going to work within the framework of your inborn normal reflexes... making a friend of your appetite, and paying attention to it; for this is a good thing... Slim people have appetites... They know how to pay attention to them... Attractive people have appetites... They also know how to pay attention to them.

In the past, you've probably been paying attention only to half the signals from your appetite... Namely, the signal that says..."Eat, I'm hungry"... But from now on, you are going to make a friend of your appetite... You will listen to your appetite advice and what your appetite is saying to you... When it says "I'm hungry,"...you will eat healthy, nutritious, and scrumptious foods...you will notice right away when the hunger feeling first disappears... and you will notice that your appetite is saying, "I'm satisfied"...and your body will automatically stop eating... You will stop eating long before you're full...because once you have a full sensation...it actually means that you have grossly overeaten... You should never want to feel full again...just satisfied...

You will restore your normal reflexes, which will keep you satisfied and bring that wonderful feeling of well-being into play... Hypnosis brings about satisfaction, which leads to relaxation, a slim, healthy, attractive body, a relaxed mind and a satiated spirit... The old urge to diet is now completely removed from your mind...for now you realize that the real answer is restoring normal body reflexes...

You will concentrate on normal body reflexes...obeying every signal... the hypnotic suggestions you receive will rapidly bring about a change necessary to ensure a permanently slim, healthy, and attractive body, which you so desire...You will find each time you are tempted to eat or drink anything that you know is wrong for you... you will easily say "no thank you" and stick by it...because the rewards of becoming slimmer and healthier are more important to you than eating the wrong and fattening foods...definitely, the rewards of being slender, more desirable, and sexier...are more important to you than eating foods that you know are wrong for you...

As you are listening to me speak, you are going deeper and deeper into relaxation... deeper and deeper down with every breath you exhale...you have noticed all the sounds have faded away in the distance...paying attention only to the sound of my voice, listening carefully to the suggestions that I am about to give you...

One thing is very important for you...you are not only going to lose weight but are permanently going to keep it off... This program is designed so that you will permanently lose all your fat... and become a lean, alert and vigorous person... You will lose all your extra weight and keep it off easily and comfortably... That means that you are going to be completely reconditioned... You will be improving your body to a new and more lean form...remember, every cell in your body changes at least once every seven years...your cells on your palms, every two hours and in your liver, every six weeks, and so forth...every new cell will be so healthy and sparkling with energy...with your new eating habits. ..

Not only will you have these new eating habits...but you will be content and happy with yourself and these new heating habits... You are going to enjoy life... eating the way nature intended...eating only when you have a real need to...for nourishment from the food you are eating...and never eating again just because you are bored or stressed out... not only now, but for the rest of your life...

In the past, you ate more than your body needed for its energy requirements...you know this is true because you ended up storing this extra energy as inert fat and gained weight...Now to lose weight and reduce this inert fat, you must burn the excess fat up... while you meet your daily requirements for energy... You will eat fewer calories than you burn each day... Later, when you are lean, you will eat only the amount you need for your physical needs each day... But for right now, you are developing habits to eat less than you're using up... We are not giving you a measured diet, for that amount will vary daily and depend greatly on your physical activities...

You will eat less than you need...for the storage already in your body will make up the difference... This may notice that eating a bit less will cause you no trouble or inconvenience...for the inert fat will be burned, and you will quickly and safely lose weight... You are naturally going to eat a great deal less than you are used to eating in the past...but it will be enough to satisfy you...because healthy nutritional foods are what your body is craving in the first place...You will eat less, and you will feel full and satisfied...finally, your body will be happy from the nutrients it is receiving... every time you take a bite from now on...when you are hungry, you will eat what the body needs and your excess fat will be used up, and both body and mind will be harmonious...

You will easily use any of your stored fat to supply extra energy to your body as it transitions to eating less and less...as you lose weight...you will naturally not need to eat as much since there is not as much of you to feed...As you eliminate the excess, you will eat far less than you need each day... for the extra calories are coming from the food you ate yesterday and last year...You will eat nothing more to replace these stored fat cells...you want them to be gone forever...

Nothing and no one can force you to overeat food or the wrong types of foods or liquids that will replace this ugly fat... you will simply say no thank you and walk away if need be...For you will never need to store fat again... Knowing that you don't want this fat ever to be replaced... These stored fat cells are gone forever... You know they were burdensome and harmful to you... and you need to get rid of them...just as an overloaded glass needs to get rid of excess liquid by spilling over...your body now releases any excess by not eating it in the first place...

No longer will you need to eat more food for this storage... You will only eat small amounts until you have used all of this stored energy, and all those ugly storehouses of fat are gone...From this moment on, you will eat less...but move more and more lively and be more and more active... for you will feel better than you have ever felt before... You lose the desire for all but a small amount of food until your weight has come down to the lean size you want... Then you will always eat sensibly and correctly for the rest of your life...

You will notice that after you change your chemistry... you have adjusted your whole body and your overall feeling to that of a wonderful sense of well-being you have... You will eat sensibly, get plenty of exercise... drink adequate liquids always to make you feel healthy, lean, trim, and desirable...

You are easily losing weight steadily every day... You are slim and shapely... The excess weight is melting off you... just melting away and disappearing... You are happy to know that you have a stronger feeling every day that you completely control your eating habits... Your mind already has a picture of yourself the way you are going... slim and shapely and sexy... It does not matter what you look like at this moment... your mind knows what it will look like after you are at your healthy weight... your mind likes this new game of using up the excess fat stored in it to mold and shape you into the new you...

New sparkling cells which make up your legs...ankles, calves and thighs...slender...shapely...fit and strong...some may call them sexy...and you body...skinny...slender waist...with just the right amount of curves for you...breasts that are just right...just the way they look in mind that is better...for a woman, lifted, firm and beautiful...for a man, formed just right...your arms, neck and face...all the new cells are formed just right...the texture...elasticity...and collagen...healthy...glowing cells...making up this new fit body of yours...
Now just relax and let all these suggestions take complete and thorough effect upon you...your mind, body, and spirit...as your subconscious mind corrects your hypothalamus to change your body's chemistry automatically... Let the monitor of your subconscious mind influence the hypothalamus to make these favorable body changes... Let your appetite control center be safely reduced so that excess fat storage will be utilized by excretion and burning of stored energy...

Eliminating all that extra harmful fat...forever...

Five minutes later

...Wonderful... All these suggestions I have given you are now reinforced...and every time you take a breath, in and out... will reinforce this...in and out...new sparkling, healthy cells...happy...rejuvenated, and ready to shine...

Take a deep breath and wiggle your toes and fingers...coming back to this moment...feeling empowered and in control of your body and weight forever...

Weight Reduction Script #2

Induction of your choice...

Although sometimes we are quite fearful of change or something new... we are well aware that there is no chance for improvement unless there is change... If we have had difficulty in some areas, we must change the old patterns... So today, I suggest we do something entirely different from what we usually do... Something that may be quite new to you... Although you have likely done it sometime in the past... Today I propose that you let yourself see yourself in a new perspective... See yourself as others might see you or as you might be seen in history...

When you are away from yourself, even for a few moments...you begin to see yourself in an entirely different light... Temporarily, if you separate yourself in time and physical distance... you can see yourself not only as you are at the moment...but as you were yesterday or even far back in childhood... You can see yourself proceeding through all the stages of growth to the present time... and even projecting your view of yourself into the future...

You are capable of doing this... It is a safe procedure... it is possible because your subconscious mind calculates time and distance differently from the subconscious mind... In the conscious mind, everything is very concrete...real... The minutes progress in an orderly fashion... to form hours, days, weeks and years... The subconscious mind works very differently... You live in the present... but if you are suddenly incredibly stressed, you call forth experiences from the past... Your natural defenses and reactions of today will respond instead to the similar stresses of last year or five years ago...

In other words...in the subconscious mind... your frame of reference is entirely different... You can be in the present... but if something provokes or excites you... in a fraction of a second, you can revert to childish or immature behavior... and relive an incident with all the sound, fury, and emotion you had the first time you experienced it... In other words, in a fraction of a second, you can span the years and relive an incident as vividly as you did the first time...

In exactly the same way, you can see some of the future... Seeing yourself as you might behave a year or five years from now... Predicting the future is possible because the attitudes you hold about yourself determine your behavior... the friends you choose, and the situations you create...Even though you may not be able to fill in other people's names or the precise location... you can predict the kind of situation you will place yourself into because of the attitudes you hold about yourself... Time and place in the subconscious mind are only relative... Your attitude and defenses remain almost unchangeable, and they interact with the environment in very much the same way throughout your life...

You can quite easily project yourself temporarily outside your body as if you were a third person... and look back at yourself and your surroundings free from the usual physical limitations... It is very safe to project yourself in spirit, out and beyond your normal physical limitations... so you can look back at yourself and understand exactly where you are... This projection is entirely under your control... You will find it relatively easy to separate much of your spirit and intellect from your body... so that you can momentarily be free from your body's limitations... From this vantage point... you can see yourself in prospective from birth to the present moment... You will become acutely aware of the minds program you had to adapt to keep your physical body alive in a world that may have seemed so threatening... You will be able to understand your family's interactions with you as you have never before been able to understand...

Best of all... from this detached, safe vantage point... you can plainly see the defenses you needed when you were tiny... You have now outgrown them just as you have outgrown the need for nursing bottles and diapers...

The projection experience... is familiar to anyone who dreams... for dreams change all the usual limitations of time and space... A good example is awakening abruptly from a very sound sleep... and being momentarily confused about where you are...

Or the perspective of a photograph...you may notice things about yourself that you do not usually notice...for in this perspective, you are looking at all of you...just like someone else does...not just from inside your mind...

You may have had the experience of looking in a three-way mirror in a clothing store, seeing yourself in profile and back view, and getting an entirely different perspective of yourself... Another way to get a projection of yourself is to look into a mirror that shows your reflection in another mirror... Then, by changing the angle slightly... you can see one mirror reflecting in another in a whole row of mirrors... almost on to eternity...

Now imagine... you in a photograph of yourself...in the same pose...but each at different ages of your life...just like a row of mirrors...but in each mirror is a different aged you...past...present...and if you like future...You line them up so that you see yourself in these mirrors at all ages, from infancy to the current time... Depending on the angle of the mirrors, you can see yourself projected either into the past or into the future...

Now picture yourself intellectually outside your own body... with a clear view of your whole life in perspective... You have in your possession all of the wisdom... all the learning... and all the understanding... that you have ever gained... In this position, you can now influence your destiny by re-programming and upgrading your attitude and defenses... You let yourself change wherever you see the need... for growth and maturity... so all your reactions may come up to your expectations as you relinquish your hang-ups...

Hear yourself encourage your whole being... to accept yourself... and approve of what you do... Especially see yourself reinforcing the normal eating patterns... to eat only when you are hungry... to see that your appetite is easily satisfied... Picture yourself enjoying food immensely ...but only in quantities you need to fulfill normal physical requirements... See yourself overcoming the temptation to eat any extra food... As you observe yourself, it becomes easier and easier to pass up unneeded food and drink... Especially note... carefully... how your need to seek approval from everyone else is disappearing... very quickly and progressively... More and more, you are approving of what you do...

See yourself also using self-hypnosis... as a very powerful and safe force for you... Its effectiveness increases... as you let part of yourself be projected beyond your usual body limitations... so that you can give yourself suggestions much more effectively as if you were a third person... Again and again, you accept the suggestion that you eat only when you truly need food and are satisfied with basic nutrition... See yourself being increasingly happy with your eating pattern... and showing approval of what you do...

You see, you have not really been paying attention to your appetite at all... because your eating has been driven by emotions rather than hunger... Eating is always proper when your appetite says, "I'm hungry"... But you've been eating even when you've not been hungry... You've been eating out of habit... even when your body had no physical need for food... You've been eating to satisfy psychological and emotional cravings... You forgot in the past to pay attention to your appetite when it says, "I'm done... I'm satisfied... Stop eating,"... From now on you will tune in on your body's sensations...

You must eat for your physical needs only... otherwise you bring into play an old instinct for self-preservation...and hoarding...which results in fat...ugly fat...please...you do not need to store fat...you are going to eat soon...remind your body of this...it is not like you are in a war and do not know when your next meal is...the fridge...grocery store is right there... You must develop the habit now... that you're always going to eat all you need... Under hypnosis, you can reinforce the normal feedback mechanisms... the checks and balances that tell you when you need food... and when your appetite is satisfied...

However strong this hypnosis may be... it cannot overcome basic survival instincts... A strong instinct is a self-preservation... Surprisingly, your concern about being overweight has probably led to sporadic dieting... This, in turn, suggests starvation... Starvation... in turn... demands defense... It brings out the instinct of self-survival... This instinct is responsible for maintaining your excess weight... Slim people eat all they want...whenever they want...

Slim people do well... Slim, attractive people say, "I eat all I want and stay the same weight."

Visualize yourself as this slim... attractive person... the slim, healthy, attractive person that you soon will be... You will soon be saying the very same thing... As you begin to talk and act like a slim, healthy, attractive person... you will quickly become one... Being overweight... is primarily not a dietary problem... but an emotional problem... You must resolve this right now...to give up yo-yo dieting forever... today you will form a new habit pattern... to eat all the healthy food you need... when your body needs it... Paying attention to your appetite... trusting your own reflexes... reinforcing the sensation...reflexes, and feedback patterns...

This is true... even though you may seem to lose the weight very slowly at first... The excess fat will be burned away in due time... You are going to be slim, healthy, and attractive... you may even have weeks where you gain a couple of pounds...don't be worried...it is all okay...your body is just going through the self-preservation...and hoarding stage...it may feel like you are dieting and not feeding it...the memory of not having enough food from an old diet you tried many years ago ...those pounds are trying to decide to stay or leave...the body is scared. You need to tell your body that it is okay...it can let go of those fat cells...you do not need to store any of that excess weight now...you have all the food you need...all the healthy food the body craves...and you will be replacing those fat cells with healthy new cells...which will give the body even more energy than it had before...You will feel wonderful in every way...tell the body right now that it is okay to let go of those old cells...it is time...and new clean, healthy, lively cells are waiting to be replaced...

By its very nature, fat contains an extremely big amount of stored energy... So, if you burn a little of it each day... you will lose only a little weight each day... Nature designed the fat stores to last a long time, so the weight loss must be gradual... but it needs to be consistent... It matters not how long it takes to gain lean proportions...the new slim and trim body... for you will surely get there... and permanently stay there... as long as you permanently rearrange your thoughts about eating... and your emotions about food... The important thing is that you have changed your habits forever... Remembering a loss of one to four pounds a week is ideal... When your excess weight is off... it is off for good... You're a new person... about to emerge from a cocoon padded with fat... Be happy with your new form... Emerge as a new person with thoroughly changed ideas and... thoroughly revised image of yourself...

Relax and let all of these suggestions sink into the deepest part of your mind's eye as an image... This image is of good and wonderful food... Food you like... There is plenty of it all around you...There always will be plenty of it... For you, there will always be enough food... You will never have to worry about starving... For you, there is plenty of food everywhere... With all this food readily available... you will never need to store any more food inside your body... There is plenty of food... plenty of the right kinds of food... all the kinds and varieties that your body needs...and when it needs it...

From now on, you will eat only the very things your body needs... one day at a time... You are through with storing fat... For you to store fat... is just as unnecessary as for you to learn to shoe horses... or make soap for the family... Fat is an extra burden on your heart and organs... Fat keeps you unhealthy... Fat can ruin and shorten your life... There is plenty of food all around you... You never again need to store food in your body...never need to store more than your body needs to use up before your next meal...which may be only a couple minutes or hours from now...

 In case you did not know or forgot...there is a small area in the central part of your brain that regulates the biochemistry of your body...and it controls the amount of fat you store in your body... This control is located in the hypothalamic area of the brain... Through the hypothalamus, your subconscious mind controls your weight by changing the body's chemistry... Hypnosis can influence your subconscious mind to alter the control of your appetite and food storage in the form of fat...

Now while under the influence of hypnosis... I suggest that you change your body's chemistry to break up these large storage houses of fat... and prevent the recurrence of new and unneeded storages of fat... ugly fat... Fat that has been putting an extra burden and overload on your body's machinery... your body will now break up and eliminate the unneeded fat stores forever... Change fat to energy and burn it up... getting rid of it by excreting it... Get rid of it through your bowels... Get rid of it in every way possible...Body, mind, and spirit... It mobilizes quite readily and you can envision the fat melting as you use it... and excrete it... The globules of fat storage are leaving the normal cells and being cleansed away... The fat is being burned up and excreted...

So as you retune your hypothalamus... you notice that your body only wants to eat at the slim body weight you envision...each day, your appetite is a little less... until you reach your ideal weight...the slim weight, slim body...that sexy body that you desire...

Take a deep breath and release all those unneeded fat cells...allowing the hypothalamus to be reprogrammed for this new desired size...your hypothalamus will be programmed to only eat the amount needed for your new weight...

When you are about in your normal day... every time you see food...you may or may not be hungry for it...but only you will know when it is the right time to eat... and how much you will eat...

Your hypothalamus is now set at this new slim body...and will trigger many times a day...at all your usual times...and send the new message out to the rest of your body...to eat and be healthy at this new weight...and you notice the changes very quickly...eating all that you need to sustain that beautiful new you...

Take a deep breath... come back to the moment... wiggle your toes and fingers...and when you are ready, open your eyes...feeling great and a little bit different than before...different because your hypothalamus has been set at the new slim you...ready to do its job and regulate your food intake...enjoy the new healthy you...

BONUS

Hypnotherapy Sample Form

Hypnotherapy

Clients Name: _____ Clients Signature _____

Date: _____ Phone Number_____
Address: _____City:_____P/C_____
Birth date (Month):_____ Practitioner: _____

1. How are you feeling today? _____   4. Have you had this type or similar session before? No / Yes
2. In your opinion are you stressed? _____   5. Any other health concerns? _____
3. Are you under going any other therapies? _____   6. What are your expectations for this session? _____

Step 1- Issue or Goal
_____
_____
_____

Step 2– Induction used   circle
Breath Spot Internalization   Count Fascination   Fractionation   Confusion   Quick   Other:
_____

Step 3– Safe place
_____
_____

Step 4– Core issue
_____

Step 5– Desired Outcome
_____

Step 6– Steps taken to achieve desired outcome:
Release of negativity or what is holding the outcome from happening
_____
_____
_____

Step 7– Post Hypnotic suggestion used No___ Yes ___
_____

Step 8 - Homework Yes ___ No ___ What
_____

Step 9 Need another session No ___ Yes ___
When _____

Step 10– Termination used:
_____

Any other FINDINGS AND COMMENTS:
_____
_____
_____
_____
_____
_____

Emotional Clearing Technique (ECT)

The Emotional Clearing Technique is designed essentially to find where in the person's body:

- They are holding the issue and emotion (dis-ease)
- When the issue first began (origin)
- Whose issue is it that is holding them back from success, emotionally, spiritually, mentally, or physically and
- How to release it.

This technique can pinpoint when the person began creating the issue. It is beneficial to know the original time when the issue started so that the brain (neurons) can release the negative emotions attached to that time frame. Your memories are stored in the Hypothalamus / limbic center of the brain and, until told to delete, will hold on forever.

Patterns are created like a habit. A person repeats a situation repeatedly, creating a pattern or negative habit. Many holistic counselors believe that this negative pattern is repeated for the person to learn a lesson and move forward. Though many people never learn the lesson and just keep reinforcing the negative emotion instead.

It is proven that we will act out the emotion that we had when the original traumatic (negative) experience happened. Meaning you will act out the feelings of whatever age you were when it happened. Ever seen a fifty-year-old act like a ten-year-old? Funny when you think about it how many people do not act their age when they are upset. E.g., Let's say, at the age of forty-five, a similar situation brings back the trauma or bad feelings of when it originally happened at the age of four. Our emotions and reactions would be like a four-year-old at any age until the person clears the emotional issue.

People usually remember either something unbelievably bad or something exceptionally good. The majority of people live their lives by how they feel. And usually will avoid anything that makes them feel bad. Then depending on what order we place, our values and morals will determine how fast we will change a bad feeling. E.g., Ted wants a new job and has been thinking about it for a few months. He knows he could eventually find a job with better pay which would make him happier. The problem is he lives paycheck to paycheck and has three kids and a wife who depends on his paychecks to pay all the bills. They could never afford him to quit and take time to find a new job. His morals of making sure his family is taken care of will win out, and his personal feelings will get stored away in his body.

Depending on how bad the feelings/regrets become will determine when a person decides to change, or it is made by karmic change (laws of the universe).
One day Ted ends up hurting himself playing with the kids and is now off work for a few weeks. His bills get behind because of loss of pay, and depending on how

severe the injury is, he may now be left with scars or sore muscles for life.

He could have taken a week off to find a new job. But the laws of the universe (you create what you think) take over.

People need (want, wish, dream, desire, etc.) many things in life. The excuses they use to avoid getting them are from one extreme to another. 'My parents would never allow that,' 'What would the neighbors think,' ' My spouse will kill me for that,' 'I can't do that.'

We are a product of our surroundings. What we believe we will manifest. If you think you are a terrible person, you will be correct. If you think you are a good person, you will be correct.

The big secret is...we cannot change others; **we can only change ourselves**. If a person does not like apple pie, it will never matter who made the apple pie, they will still not like it. The emotion is embedded in the mind, and until the origin and truth of why they do not like apple pie is found, the person cannot change the feeling.

Negative feelings take up way too much time and energy for a person to hold on to.

What happens to a man
Is less significant than
What happens within.

This is where ECT comes in, and as a practitioner, we can help the person find out why they do not like apple pie or whatever it is they want to change about themselves.

ECT will assist the practitioner when a person comes in and asks for help in:
Finding out why they have an issue
Why they cannot get better or achieve a goal in their life
Ideas on how to clear it up.

Energy Clearing Technique has eight steps.
Steps 1-6 will tell you what, where, age, and whose issue it is. Step 7 tells you which way to help clear the issue. Step 8 will tell you if the issue is complete and if they need another session.

You will need a method of determining the answers:
Body pendulum, pendulum, finger, or arm testing knowledge works to perform this technique.

WHAT IS MUSCLE TESTING?

From my Secrets of a Healer- Magic of Muscle Testing book,

Muscle testing is a technique that healthcare professionals have used for many years to evaluate the function and effectiveness of the muscles.

In traditional Chinese Medicine, the body is considered a whole being. Man is understood as a structural, chemical, mental, and spiritual being.

HOW TO TEST?

There are two methods to choose from when you muscle test your person. Five if you know how to use a pendulum.

TESTING METHOD #1: MUSCLE TEST THE ARM

Practitioner, what to do to train the person's arm:
Hold the (left or right) arm straight out in front (or out to the side) and parallel to the floor.
Demonstrate a 'yes' by asking them to "hold" (the arm should be firm, not held with all his might but just a solid, straight arm parallel to the floor).
Demonstrate a 'no' by asking them to let the arm lower to the side of the body.
Show them three times what a yes and no are (you may have to hold his arm up for yes and move his arm down

to the side for no. What you are doing is training/programming the mind.

Once the person understands the process, you test the arm; with your two fingers flat above the wrist bone press with 2 pounds of pressure
with a 2-inch movement
for 2 seconds on the extended arm, saying, "Arm firm means yes."

Now say, "Arm down is no" (while you press with your two fingers flat above the wrist bone, with 2 pounds of pressure, with a 2-inch movement, for 2 seconds on the extended arm). The arm should have dropped/lowered to the side of the body.

Do this action of yes/on and no/off about three times each. You are programming the person's mind to be able to answer you.

It may take you quite a few times to learn the pressure and to notice the arm being strong, not letting go for a 'yes' and let go, dropping to the side for a 'no.' The thinking of some persons gets in the way so much that you may have to train them a few times or teach them body pendulum.

TESTING METHOD #2: BODY PENDULUM:

Have the person stand upright.
- Have the person lean forward from the ankles saying, "Forward is a 'yes,' without falling" (the person needs to remain stiff, like a board).
- Have the person lean backward from the ankles saying, "Backward is a 'no,' without falling."
- Have the person repeat this movement back and forward three times to program the mind.

YOU CAN ALSO USE A PENDULUM

Emotional Clearing Procedure:

There are eight steps to this procedure.

Step one-   Issue

Step two-   Chakra

Step three-   Meridian/Organ

Step four-   Emotion

Step five-   Age

Step six-   What or Whom

Step seven-   Release Emotion / Issue

Step eight-   Finish

STEP ONE:
Issue

Have the person <u>think</u> of the *issue or a goal they want to achieve.*

> This is a problem they want to fix or clear up. When you write the problem on paper, ensure it is clear and detailed.
>
> If the person doesn't have one, just have them say out loud, "The most important issue at this time."

STEP TWO:
Chakra

While the person is thinking about the issue.

Pendulum or muscle test which of the seven *Chakras* is off-balance: **Stop on the first one that muscle tests yes!**

(The first <u>one</u> that says 'yes' is the answer).

Name of Chakra	AKA *(also known as)*
1. Root	/ Base / Muladhara
2. Sacral	/ Sex / Svadhisthana
3. Solar Plexus	/ Navel / Manipura
4. Heart	/ Anahata
5. Throat	/ Vishuddha
6. Brow	/ Third Eye / Ajna
7. Crown	/ Sahaswara

STEP THREE:

Meridian / Organ

From the answer to <u>step two</u>, and while the person is thinking about the issue, pendulum or muscle test which Meridian/Organ in that specific Chakra *needs balancing*. *Chakras have more than one Meridian, test which <u>one</u> is the catalyst (the main one).

1. Root / Base / Muladhara Chakra
   Meridian/Organ: One of these four:

   1) Kidney *(right)*,

   2) Large Intestine,

   3) Anus/Rectum,

   4) Adrenal *(part of triple warmer/sanjiao)*

2. Sacral Chakra / Sex / Svadhisthana
   Meridian/Organ: One of these four:

   1) Kidney *(left)*,

   2) Prostrate

   3) Uterus

   4) Testes/Ovaries

3. Solar Plexus / Navel / Manipura Chakra
   Meridian/Organ: One of these four:

    1) Stomach/Spleen/Pancreas

    2) Liver/Gall bladder

    3) Small Intestine

    4) Pancreas

4. Heart / Anahata Chakra
   Meridian/Organ: One of these three:

    1) Heart

    2) Lung (chen)

    3) Thymus/Immunity

5. Throat / Vishuddha Chakra
   Meridian/Organ: One of these four:

    1) Throat

    2) Speech Organs

    3) Lungs (volume voice)

    4) Thyroid *(part of triple warmer/sanjiao)*

6. Brow / Third Eye / Ajna Chakra
   Meridian/Organ: One of these four:

   1) Hindbrain

   2) Midbrain

   3) Eyes

   4) Pituitary *(part of triple warmer/sanjiao)*

7. Crown / Sahaswara Chakra
   Meridian/Organ: One of these four:

   1) Neo-cortex

   2) Pineal

   3) Central / Ren

   4) Governing / Du

STEP FOUR:

Emotion

From the answer of <u>step three</u>, and while the person is thinking about the issue, pendulum or muscle test which *Emotion* (only one) under the Meridian/Organ from step three.

1) Root/Base/Muladhara Chakra
Confidence & Courage / Fear & Insecurity

Kidney (right) Bladder	Large Intestine	Anus/Rectum	Adrenal
Fear	Guilt	Releasing	Defeatism
Anxiety	Grief	Dumping	Not caring for self
Peace	Regret	Anger to release	Anxiety
Dread	Release	Holding on to the garbage	Sense of safety
Terror	Self-worth	Quilt	Lack of physical energy
Panic	Enthusiasm	Remorse	Heaviness
Frustration	Depression	Not feeling good enough	Balance
Impatience	Indifference	Desire for punishment	Worry
Inner Direction	Compassion	Ungrounded	Fretfulness

Confidence	Fear of letting go	Clearing	Fear
Indecisive	Holding on to past	Leaving	Energy
Pissed off	Stability	Abandoning	Power
Fear of letting go	Apathy	Discarding	Strength
Holding on to old ideas	Responsibility	Keeping	Intensity
Phobia	Blame	Staying	Weakness
Paranoia	Relief	Backup	Exhausted
Cautious	Freedom	Goodbye	Drained

2) Sacral/Sex/Svadhisthana Chakra
Love, Truth & Self-respect / Unfulfilled Lust & Negative feelings

Kidney (*left*)	Prostrate	Uterus	Testes/Ovaries
Fear	Masculine	Home of creativity	Creation
Anxiety	No Strength	Home issues	Life
Phobia	Sexual guilt	Hysteria	Creative blocks
Fire of Life	Sexually pressured	Relaxation	Intimacy issues
Untrustworthy	Belief in aging	Stubbornness	Dislike change
Source	Fear of masculinity	Safety	Desire
Foundation	Gloomy	Protection	Remorse
Starting Point	Sensual	Well-being	Invention

3) Solar Plexus/ Navel/Manipura Chakra
Self-worthiness / Pride, Anger & Unworthiness

Stomach/ Spleen/ Pancreas	Liver/ Gall bladder	Small Intestine	Pancreas
Unreliable	Content	Hurting	Sweetness in life
Criticism	Distressed	Joyfulness	Low self-esteem
Contentment	Vengefulness	Traumatized	Delight
Disappointment	Resentment	Sorrow	Happy
Deprived	Self-righteous	Unappreciated	Bored
Nausea	Transformation	Anxiety	Energy
Greed	Responsibility	Hyper	Pleasure
Empty	Unhappiness	Discouraged	Enjoyment
Sympathy	Irritability	Nourishing	Bliss
Empathy	Hostility	Sadness	Sadness
Harmony	Anger	Apathy	Harmony
Disgust	Rage	Shock	Lovability
Hungry for more	Condemning	Assimilation	Appeal
Craving Sweetness	Bitterness	Nervousness	Friendliness
Obsessions	Pride	Blocked	Coherence
Unfulfilled	Ego	Accommodating	Discord
Fear of the new	Personal power	Indigestion	Need More
Dread	Ambition	Congested	Misery

Fear of rejection	Lack of Willpower	Obstruction	Ecstasy
Inability to assimilate the new	Nasty	Hindered	Overindulge

4) Heart/Anahata Chakra
Universal love / Possessive Romance, Fell, Loss, Grief, Hurt & Jealousy

Heart	Lung (chen)	Thymus/Immunity
Forgiveness	Cheerful	Feeling attacked
Empathy	Regret	They are out to get me
Self-confidence	Snooty	Balance
Self-respect	Humble	Sickness
Confidence	Modesty	Energetic
Self-conscious	Sincerity	Tired
Insecure	Hopelessness	Can't go on
Security	Intolerance	Feed up
Mad	Injustice	Stifled
Hate	Grief	Subdued
Love	Fear to take life in	Smothered
Lack of joy	Depression	Chocked
Relationships	Worthy	Suppressed
Compassion	Life is a Burden	Spirited
Self-doubt	Holding Back	Vitality

5) Throat/Vishuddha Chakra
The exultation of freedom of speech / Frustration of expression

Throat	Speech Organs	Lungs (volume voice)	Thyroid
Lack of Creativity	Self-expression	Always Yelling	Humiliation
Swallowed anger	Communication	Loud	When my turn
Refusal to change	Manifestation	Integrity	I never get to do what I want
Difficulty speaking your truth	Utterance	Noisy	Shame
Expression	Speaking Tongues	Deafening	Embarrassment
Openness	Lectured	Shrill	Dishonor
Truth	Statement	Load mouthed	Dignity

6) Brow/Third Eye/Ajna Chakra
Clarity, Intuition & Understanding / Confusion

Hindbrain	Midbrain	Eyes	Pituitary
Survival	Emotions	Fear of seeing past, present future issues	Despair
Basic needs	Feelings	Not liking what is seen	Unhappy
Reproduction	Memories	Fear of seeing self	Lightness
Poor Intuition	Self-reflection	Not wanting to see	Heaviness
Difficulty making decisions	Lack of inspiration	Clarity	Loneliness
Endurance	Reminiscence	Lucidity	Humiliated
Death	Recollections	Transparency	Balance
Existence	Recall	Luminousness	Buoyancy
Fight or Flight	Celebration	Brightness	Control

7) Crown / Sahaswara Chakra
Permanent, Easy without effort & Happiness / Satisfaction & Despair

Neo-cortex	Pineal	Central / Ren	Governing / Du
Beliefs	Spirituality	Overwhelm	Embarrassing
Stubborn	Connection to God	Shyness	Unsupported
Refuse to change	Difficult Meditating	Success	(Dis) honesty
Self-knowledge	Holiness	Shame	(Dis) trust
Aimlessness	Mysticism	Self-respect	Truth
Principles	Magical	Control	Got Your Back
Views	Supernatural	Balanced	Reality
Ideas	Religious Beliefs	Devastated	Facts
Inspiration	Faith	Dishonor	Genuineness

STEP FIVE:

Age

Pendulum or muscle test the *age* that this <u>issue</u> (step one) happened at /originated.

You need the exact age.

A) This Life -   (Once you find the five years, find the exact age)

- Conception to birth
- Birth to 5
- 6 to 10
- 11 to 15
- 16 to 20
- 21 to 25
- 26 to 30
- 31 to 35
- 36 to 40
- 41 to 45
- (to today's age)

STEP SIX:

What or Whom

Pendulum or muscle test – *Whom or what* did this issue originate from?

Pick only one A-E and then pick one in the category.

A) Person

- ○ From yourself?
- ○ Friends? — Male / Female? (Think about the person and test to make sure)
- ○ Family? — Male / Female?
- ○ Co-workers? — Male / Female?
- ○ Enemy?
- ○ Animal?
- ○ Other (think of something else)

B) Place

1. House?
2. City /Town?
3. Province?
4. Country?
5. Continent?
6. World?
7. Other?

C) Thing

1. Money?
2. Items?

3. God?
4. Religion?
5. Other?

D) Event

1. Birthday?
2. Holiday?
3. Christmas?
4. Wedding?
5. Funeral?
6. Other?

E) If it is not A-D, then think of anything else that comes to mind.

STEP SEVEN:

1st Muscle Test the state of well-being, balance those needed.

- Physical,
- Emotional,
- Mental
- Spiritual

2nd Muscle Test the appropriate choice of Balance Idea

These are just some IDEAS (there are thousands of ways to balance)

*** You can only do the <u>ones you know how to do.</u> <u>T</u>here are many ideas here.

#1) Color:

> Test each <u>Chakra</u> to see which ones are off. Have the seven color samples 5" x 5" squares, now starting from the crown down, and have the person see the color and think about the color for a few moments. Then show the next color of the Chakra colors that were "off."

> <u>Chakra & Color</u>

> 1) Root / Base / Muladhara - red

> 2) Sacral / Sex / Svadhisthana - orange

> 3) Navel / Solar Plexus / Manipura - yellow

> 4) Heart / Anahata - green, pink

5) Throat / Vishuddha - light blue

6) Brow/ Ajna - indigo

7) Crown / Sahaswara - violet, white, gold

Idea #2) Chakra balances with pendulum:

Hold the pendulum above the crown Chakra and allow the pendulum to spin in any direction that it wants to, this will correct the Chakra (if needed) and balance it. My intent while holding the pendulum is to balance the Chakra allowing the pendulum to move in any direction needed for balancing. Once the pendulum stops moving, move on to the brow Chakra and repeat. Continue the same procedure on all the Chakras.

Idea #3) Balance with sound (four choices):

Sound Therapy

	Note	Mantra	Scale	Hertz
1)	C	LAM	Do	396hz
2)	D	VAM	Ra	417hz
3)	E	RAM	Mi	528hz
4)	F	YAM	Fa	639hz
5)	G	HAM	So	741hz
6)	A	KSHAM	La	852hz
7)	B	AUM /OM	Ti	963hz

Idea #4) Crystal or Tibetan Bowls, Music, Tuning Forks, etc.
To balance, play the appropriate Chakra sound for the Chakra that was muscle tested in Step #2.

Idea #5) Healing Stone Balance:

Test each Chakra to see which ones are off.
Place the appropriate stone on the person's body where the Chakra is for 10 minutes to overnight, to carry with them for __ days (muscle test how long it is needed).

Healing Stones

(Pick one of the stones from the list for the Chakra tested in Step #2)

1) Red jasper, Agate, Bloodstone, Garnet, Ruby, Smoky quartz

2) Carnelian, Moonstone, Tourmaline

3) Citrine, Amber, Tiger's eye, Yellow Topaz, Agate

4) Aventurine, Emerald, Green jade, Rose quartz, Kunzite

5) Blue lace agate, Aquamarine, Turquoise, Chalcedony

6) Sodalite, Lapis Lazuli, Opal

7) Amethyst, Crystal, Topaz, Alexandrite, Sapphire

Idea #6) Aromatherapy
***_Check contra-indications of oils_**

For the Chakra from Step #2. (Muscle test which oil is needed).

Have the person apply it to their body

(mix ten drops of grapeseed or olive oil with one drop of essential oil).

Place one drop on Kleenex and have them smell.

Aromatherapy

Pendulum which oil in the Chakra to use:

1) Grapefruit, Hyssop, Pine, *Cedar, *Sage, *Ylang Ylang, *Patchouli

2) Patchouli, Sage, Apple, *Sandalwood, *Lavender, *Fennel

3) Juniper, Lemon, Black Pepper, Ginger

4) *Lavender, Cedarwood, *Rose, *Sandalwood

5) Dill, Peppermint, Immortelle, *Sandalwood, *Tea tree

6) Vanilla, *Basil, Lilac, *Sandalwood, *Lavender, *Jasmine, *Eucalyptus

7) *Frankincense, Geranium, Basil, *Myrrh, *Sandalwood

(*Essential oils = Ayurveda)

Idea #7) Written

    I.   Have the person write out everything that happened and their feelings,

    II.   The next day if no more can be written, take the paper and burn it in a safe place (fireplace), take three deep breaths, and think love while you are burning the paper.

    III.   If the person can keep writing, repeat until nothing else can be added, then do step II.

Idea #8) Hug A Tree

Idea #9) Reiki / Or similar technique (Hands on Healing)

Idea #10) Muscle Testing

    Quick Fix (Neuro-Lymph points), Meridian Walking, Source Points

Idea #11) Tapping or Emotional Freedom Technique (EFT)

Idea #12) Holistic Therapy (Massage, Reflexology, Shiatsu, etc.).

Idea #13) Prayer

Idea #14) Forgiveness Release

Idea #15) Go on a Holiday, to a Movie, to a Restaurant, etc.

Idea #16) Learn Something New... take a course, read a book, attend a seminar, etc.

Idea #17) Meditation – Aka Cords, Chakra balance, Color of Energy, etc.

Idea #18) BiofeedBack

Idea #19) 100 Goals List / Bucket List

Idea #20) Neuro Linguists Programming

Idea #21) Hypnotherapy

Idea #22) Affirmations (Louise Hay) or make up your own

Idea #23) 5 Elements

Idea #24) Herbs, Nutrition, Homeopathy

Idea #25) Fitness

Idea #26) Bach Remedy, Flower Essence, Sound Essence

Idea #27) Hertz, Vibration, Auricions

Idea #28) Reversing Electromagnetic Radiation

Idea #29) Auriculotherapy (Ear Reflexology)

Idea #30) Acupressure, Acupuncture

Idea #32) One of the 5 Pillars

Idea #31) Make Up Your Own Release Idea

(Make sure to test if it will work for that person)

STEP EIGHT:

Is the Session's Issue Finished?

Pendulum or Muscle Test if the session is completed.

- o You should explain to your person that the issue is gone/finished once step 8 is successful.
  - There are times when an issue may have other issues attached to it.
    - E.g., Money may have many issues causing the person trouble—relationships, etc.
- o You may want to test how many issues or sessions are needed to clear totally.

- o With the person's permission, you can test when the person should come back for another session or have them call the next day when they aren't feeling so vulnerable.

The book *Heal Your Body by Louise Hay* is for reference to a physical problem that correlates to an emotional issue.

If you have a person telling you about a problem in their body, refer to the *Heal Your Body* book by looking up the body part alphabetically.

The book has the body part, the emotion, and an affirmation that a person can say or write to help heal the body as homework.

For more insight, at the back of the book is a picture of the spine and what nerves are connected to what body part.

ECT Sample Form

Emotional Clearing Technique

Clients Name: _____ Clients Signature _____

Date: _____ Phone Number_____

Address: _____ City: _____ P/C_____

Birth date (Month): _____ Practitioner: _____

1. How are you feeling today? _____
2. In your opinion are you stressed? _____
3. Are you under going any other therapies? _____

4. Have you had this type or similar session before? No / Yes
5. Any other health concerns? _____
6. What are your expectations for this session? _____

Step 1 - Issue
_____
_____
_____
_____

Step 2 - Chakra   _____

Step 3 - Meridian/Organ   _____

Step 4 - Emotion   _____

Step 5- Age: This Life ___ (find exact age and the day, month, year) _____

Step 6- What or Whom: Themselves _____ Family _____ Friend _____ Co-worker _____

Male: who _____ Female; who _____ Animal _____ Money _____ Items _____ God

_____ Religion _____ Event _____ Person _____ Place _____ Thing _____

Other _____

Step 7- Release Emotion: _____

Step 8 - Finished   Yes _____ No _____

Homework Yes _____ No _____ What
_____
_____

Need another session Yes _____ No _____ When
_____

Any other FINDINGS AND COMMENTS:
_____
_____
_____
_____
_____
_____
_____
_____

Practitioners Signature: _____

Guided Meditation

Hypnotherapy and Meditation differ because the person does not answer or talk to you.

MASTERING YOUR INNER GENIE MEDITATION

Get yourself ready... get yourself ready to relax...

Get yourself very comfortable... get ready to meet your inner genie... your subconscious mind...
Get ready to unlock, gain access, control, add, and to release any negative energy holding you back from your wishes, wants, dreams, and desires... When you are ready, you can close your eyes or if you prefer to keep them open, that is okay too... imagine breathing in... sparkling, vibrant creative energy... breathe out... you are releasing any negative energy you do not need into a cosmic vacuum cleaner, a cosmic garbage can...

Take a deep breath in... all the way down to your toes... releasing... cosmic garbage...

Deep breath... breathing in... and relaxing even more ... breathing out, releasing...

Three more times... breathing in...deep tummy breath... and relaxing...breathing out, releasing...

Breathing in...deep tummy breath... and relaxing... breathing out, releasing...

Wonderful... 1 more time... breathing in...deep, deep breath... and relaxing...breathing out releasing...

Allowing yourself to envision tomorrow... imagine how you would love the day to unfold... accomplishing at least one goal or task in particular... that you will complete... imagine and sense it now as if it was happening from start to finish... go ahead and imagine the goal or task being finished...

...

If you are working on any new positive habits, imagine that you are doing them now...

...

Now permit yourself to imagine having the experiences you would like to have at being successful in all aspects of your life... sense it now, imagine the life of your dreams as if it was real...

...

Next, imagine yourself in the future... an older version of yourself... however many years ahead you would like to imagine is up to you... each time you do this meditation, you can be a different age or the same age as last time... Let go and enjoy what your subconscious mind is inventing for you... let yourself go, and have fun creating and imagining...

What are you doing?

Where do you live?..

Who do you live with?..

What do you do with your day?..

Imagine asking yourself any question you like to receive more details...

What are you enjoying?..

How are you doing?..

Take notice of what you could improve on?.. It means looking back from that futuristic point in your life backward... noticing a different perspective... looking back in time because it has not happened yet... you may choose to do a 360-degree turn and notice the life in all kinds of perspectives... notice from the "I am" perspective... from your point of view...

Notice it from the "you are" perspective... how others perceive you...

Notice it from the "they are" perspective... how the masses perceive you...

Imagine floating above yourself and viewing that perspective of yourself... or if you see yourself from a bird's eye or a child's perspective looking up at you... or from a significantly older person's perspective... each perspective has a different view on life... you can do this with any area in your life, with just a different intent like... health, wealth, and happiness... relationships, career, education, business, legacy...

Creating your destiny and your dreams into reality is like growing up from a small child's perspective... curiosity, then action, then practice and more practice until it becomes ingrained and so natural that you do not even think about it anymore, it just is... it just happens... it just becomes part of your life, natural and easy...

...

Take a breath and relax... really let go... simply listen to my voice breathing deeply... feel your breath as it goes in... and as you let go, it goes all the way out... completely relaxed...

As you breathe in and out... notice a wave of calmness coming over your body as you let go... breathing in and breathing out... as you take a breath in, relax all the muscles in your feet... take a deep breath, relax, and release... all your concerns about your day... any stress, pain, anxiety just dissolve... so relaxed and comfortable that any outside noises just helps you to relax even more... a deeply relaxed state of relaxation... so relaxed that your body, mind, and soul can create the life, the ideal body, or whatever you desire, just by relaxing and imagining it to be true... focus on whatever you would like... anything you are ready to create ... simply imagine it now...

...

Take a deep relaxing breath and let the muscles in your legs, knees, and hips relax... any and all tension disappears... so relaxed that you start to notice a very positive shift beginning to take place in your being... in your energy field... a very subtle transformation... your life becomes better and better each and every day... you meet new friends, enjoy old friends. Even your family starts to notice this subtle change in your personality... you are happier, and healthier and an excess of money seems to flow into your life magically... making it easier... making it better... so relaxed, so calm, so enjoyable...

Taking your next deep breath, you relax your torso... all the muscles and organs, every cell in your body, relax and release, feeling more and more rejuvenated, younger, healthier, fresher with every breath you take... breathing in and breathing out... all this happens simply and easily by just letting go, of thoughts and care, letting go of the concerns of the day...

The power of letting go... allowing healing, vital life force energy to infuse and inspire your body, mind, and soul... all the new resources you will need for your day, your goal, and your task will be available as quickly as the oxygen you breathe, natural and automatic upon awakening... be that tomorrow morning or in a few minutes... enhancing the quality of your life... the quality of all relationships, the quality of all thoughts... nourishing and revitalizing every cell of your body... to be in tune with the power of your subconscious mind... the power of your inner genie...

Your focus... your ability to manifest your wishes, wants, dreams, and desires... becomes better and better each and every day...

Relaxing all the muscles in your neck and shoulders, relaxing your arms, hands, and fingers... breathing in and out... completely relaxed... so relaxed that each time you listen to this meditation, you go even deeper into relaxation, calmer, and upon awakening your body, mind, and soul... your confidence, your success will be improved, enhanced, enriched... it may be subtle... you may not even notice it happening... but it is there... calm, peace, happiness, success... take a deep breath in, relaxing... releasing... let all the energy out... and bringing in all that you need... creating a new set point... a new point like resetting a timer... resetting a watch... whatever you are needing, creating, focusing on... is your new set point... your new anchor...

Take a breath creating your new set point to be just the way you imagine it to be... imagine seeing it, feeling it, hearing it, and knowing that it means now... allowing it to be possible... allowing the possibility of it to be possible... allow your subconscious mind to create a new pathway, a new street, a new road to this idea... a new focus... allowing your subconscious mind to be able to create a new filing system, which stores your information even better, with easier access to this new filing system... download like you just got upgraded... like having a new computer with new software, new commands, new hardware...

Deep breath in... every cell in your body is being upgraded now... releasing all old beliefs...

Take a deep breath in, even deeper than the last... relax even more... able to access, control, and reprogram your subconscious mind as easily and naturally as brushing your teeth... take a deep breath in and relax your neck and head... all the muscles in your face... your cheeks, even your tongue relaxes... and release anything and everything holding you back from your ideal body, mind, and soul... breathing in and out...

Allowing all of this to become possible... next time you listen to this meditation and each time you listen to it... knowing you can change your path... change your goal... change your task... change your focus... change your old habits that don't serve you anymore... you can add new ideas, goals... thoughts, concepts, perceptions, beliefs, dreams, knowledge, and solutions... to your subconscious mind... new thoughts... which are even more beneficial to your body, mind, and soul... each and every day you have new opportunities that arise that you can act upon now with grace, patience, honesty, integrity, and ease... because you have the choice, the knowledge, the intelligence, the natural talents... inspiration and motivation...

Take another moment and focus on your new set point... your desired outcome...

Take a breath... notice a path... some of you have already been on this path before... if you have not already been on this path... you will find a key... pick it up and hold onto it... and for those that have already done this and picked up your key before, you know what it unlocks... go ahead of me... I will catch up with you in a bit... and for those of you for who this is the first time with this new key... it unlocks your subconscious mind... as you take your next deep breath, you instinctively already know exactly how to unlock your mind, so go ahead and use this special key to unlock your subconscious mind... notice all the amazing things your inner genie has access to...

Take note of what you need to change... to guarantee success on whatever goal or task you have chosen to work on... notice your subconscious mind is like a filing cabinet... you have access to go through the files... remembering all the good and bad experiences, lessons, and emotions... knowing you can remove any files that you no longer need or that don't serve your current purpose... go ahead imagine reading them quickly and just unconsciously knowing which ones you can remove... all out of date files and programs that hold you back from becoming the person you desire to become... these files are similar to a personal computer... they were created, they were programmed into the machine... and they can be erased and rebooted... you can organize these files into categories... keep it, toss them, and decide later category... you can color-code them or whatever your imagination comes up with... it can be almost instantaneously done for you... your inner genie can work magic with anything it can think of... anything it wants to imagine, real or pretend... your inner genie... your subconscious mind has amazing capabilities...

Notice you have a choice... you know where the files are. You can always come back and do it later...But, today, there may be 1 or 2 at least that you can do right this moment... choose to get in the habit of cleaning and removing all the old, outdated, torn, wrecked, broken, hated, disliked files and programs... that no longer serve who you are anymore... notice you have a file... quickly scan it over (you intuitively know if it is to be deleted...

or... if it is needed for another reason)... the ones that are okay to delete, go ahead and imagine burning them, pushing the delete button, shredding them, or any other way that comes to your mind to be rid of them forever... even delete the folder it was stored in...remove that too... go ahead and remove all of the out of date files and programs that no longer serve a purpose... any old beliefs, habits, patterns that no longer serve a purpose...

...

With taking your next deep breath... your subconscious mind now creates and imagines your next new idea... your next new path... or if you like, you can rototill up the dirt of the old path and start again... adding new dirt and nutrients and plant new fresh ideas and watch them grow and mature... you can imagine planting bigger plants that have already matured somewhat to be already beautiful, and not so much time is needed to wait for all the amazing benefits... a mature plant that all it needs to do is be loved and nurtured for its roots to take place and know that this new place is perfect to start growing even bigger, even better than before... creating the ideal perfect reason for its existence... because it was chosen to be there... breath in deep and let the roots be nurtured no matter what way you have chosen for this new idea, this new goal, this new task to solidify and become one within your body, mind, and soul...

... you have the power to empower yourself every day... with accomplishing your goals, finishing your tasks, and achieving your dreams... you have the ability to choose... where you go, what to do, who you spend quality time with... how to invest your money... and anything else you can imagine doing, seeing, feeling, and knowing... all that is perfect for you... you have control over your inner genie... you have control over your subconscious mind...

Take a deeply relaxing, rejuvenating breath... so excited for the changes in your life... so excited about creating your future like this... and so it is exciting to know that you can create like this... knowing this key is impossible to lose... it is like having a soul key to your existence... a magical key to unlock, gain access, control your subconscious mind... all the new books, new courses, new people, new places, new experiences... knowing now that you are in control of your inner genie... your subconscious mind... you have the power to choose to reprogram your inner genie, your subconscious mind... you are the genie... you have the magic, and there is an infinite amount and supply of wishes, dreams, wants, and desires granted...

Indefinite, limitless, unrestricted... infinite amount and supply of wishes, dreams, wants, and desires granted...

Indefinite, limitless, unrestricted... repeat in your mind... indefinite, limitless, unrestricted... infinite possibilities... infinite realities... it is my choice... indefinite, limitless, unrestricted... possibilities... granted...

With your next deep breath, you will be gifted a token, a symbol... and you will have proof in the awakened state of your being... in your day-to-day life... proof that you are on the right path... proof, evidence, verification... confirmation that this is your truth... confirmation usually comes in threes... but whatever you have decided as your token of proof will be granted... the proof, the confirmation needed... the universe has your back... you will either see your token, hear it, feel it, or just know... the sign that guides you confirms what your inner genie already knows... but now also confirms in your conscious mind, your awake state as well... that you are heading in the correct perfect direction...

...

For whatever reason, notice a feather... imagine it as real as you like... the shape... color... size... the style... imagine this feather to help solidify this new belief... from now on, when you see a feather, it will represent, calmness, serenity... peacefulness, lightness, ease, and grace... every time you see a feather... you will be reminded of this meditation, and you will know without a doubt that you are the genie... you are the creator of your destiny...

Take a breath and imagine that it is tomorrow morning... and you are waking up feeling refreshed and so alive... so ready to step into the day... knowing you are inspired, motivated, and empowered to do, see, feel, and know that you are capable, competent, knowledgeable, and successful at completing your goal... go about your day knowing you have all the pieces needed to complete your puzzle... your masterpiece... breathing in all the cosmic energy required... and exhaling out any energy that is not needed, into the cosmos... breathing in all the way down to your DNA... clear sparkling, vibrant creative energy for your emotional, physical, mental and spiritual self...breathing out...

Breathing in ... all that is needed... breathing out all that is not... knowing that it is easy to manifest the life of your dreams... breathing in... and breathing out... you do it so naturally already... breathing in the energy you need... and breathing out, all that you do not... so simple, so sweet, so easy...

One more time... breathing in all the way down to your DNA... clear sparkling, vibrant creative energy for your emotional, physical, mental, and spiritual self...

... with your next breath, you have a choice... if you are listening to this in bed, then just have an excellent night's sleep... waking up with your inner genie already knowing what it needs to do tomorrow...

If you are listening to this during the day... knowing you have the key to manifest all your dreams, wishes, wants, and desires into reality... if it is during the day, wiggle your toes coming back to the moment... if it is day time... take a breath now and be awake knowing that your body, mind, and soul knows exactly what to do to create the life of your dreams... just as easy as breathing... enjoy your day knowing you will notice your token... and if you see a feather today know that you are reminded that you are the genie...

If it is daytime, awake, wiggling your toes... breathing in and manifesting your dreams into reality...

Other Ways to Practice Self-Hypnosis/Meditation

Candle Meditation

1. Get a candle, one that can burn safely for about half an hour, and light it,
2. Get yourself comfortable, very comfortable. You will need to be able to stay in this position for half an hour,
3. Take a few deep breaths,
4. Relax,
5. Look into the candle . . . and stare into the flame,
6. Allow any thoughts or feelings to surface, just be,
7. Continue looking at the flame for the entire meditation,
8. Allow the focus of your eyes to relax, dis-focus,
9. Stare at the candle's flame for half an hour,
10. When you are finished, wiggle your toes, and take a deep breath,
11. Bring your attention back to the room, feeling refreshed and awake,
12. Write/Journal about your thoughts, feelings, and anything that you experienced.

Picture Meditation

1. Get an abstract picture, use Pinterest or something similar,
2. Get yourself comfortable, very comfortable. You will need to be able to stay in this position for half an hour,
3. Take a few deep breaths,
4. Relax,
5. Look and stare at the picture,

6. Allow any thoughts or feelings to surface, just be,
7. Continue looking at the picture for the entire meditation,
8. Allow the focus of your eyes to relax, dis-focus,
9. Stare at the picture's flame for half an hour,
10. When you are finished, wiggle your toes and take a deep breath,
11. Bring your attention back to the room, feeling totally refreshed and awake,
12. Write/Journal about your thoughts, feelings, and anything that you experienced.

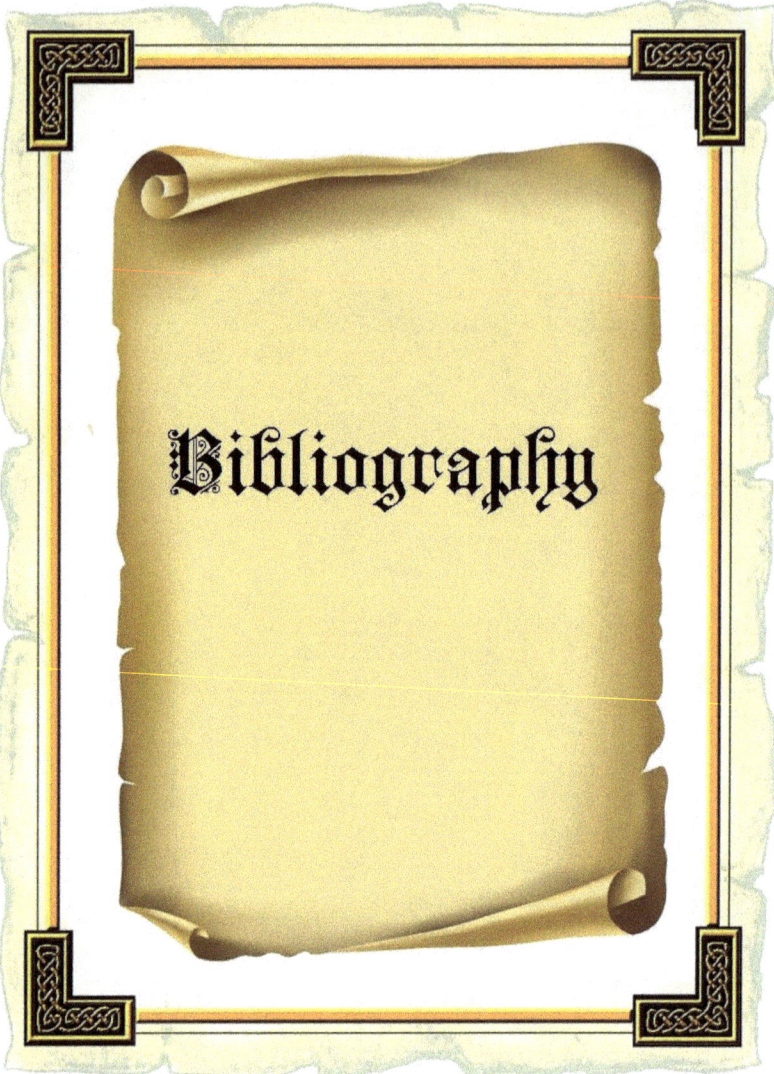

Bibliography

Bibliography

Suggested books to read:

Textbook– Prescription for Nutritional Healing ISBN 7-35918-33077-1

Textbook– Heal Your Body, by Louise Hay ISBN 0-937611-35-2

Textbook- The Definitive Book of Body Language ISBN 0-553-80472-3

Textbook– Choices, interviewing and counselling skills for Canadians ISBN 0130665851

Much of this information was taken from the course information created when I owned the Canadian Institute of Natural Health and Healing Accredited College

Bachmann, Rose Dr.

    1996   Emotional Polarity Course

Bennet Stellar University

    2005   Neuro-Linguistic Programming Course

British Columbia Institute of Holistic Studies

    2001   Advanced Aromatherapy Course

Brummet, Connie

> 2000 Canadian Institute Of Natural Health &
> Healing, ECT Course

Cameron, Julia

> 2006 The Artist's Way

Chopra, Deepak

> Ageless Body, Timeless Mind
>
> The Seven Spiritual Laws of Success: A Practical
> Guide to the Fulfillment of Your Dreams
>
> The Way of the Wizard: Twenty Spiritual Lessons
> for Creating the Life You Want

Colour Spectrums

> 2003 Introductory Session Course

Dewe, Bruce & Joan

> 1991 Five Element Emotion Chart

Gienger, Michael

> 2009 Healing Crystals: the A-Z guide to 430
> gemstones

Gray, Katherine

> 1986 Keys To Prosperity Course

Hay, Louise L.

> 1988 Heal Your Body, Hay House Publications,
> ISBN 978-0-937611-35-7

International BodyTalk Association

2009   Module 1&2 Course

Levy, L Susan and Lehr, Carol

1996   Your Body Can Talk ISBN 0-934252-68-8

McHugh, Diane

2002   Reiki Level III Course

Margaret, Ripple

2000   master's degree Reiki Course

Milton H. Erickson – Many of his books

Minckler, James

1999   Energy Balancing Course

Molloy, Brenda

2005   Table Shiatsu Course

Mulders, Evelyn

1998   Touch For Health Levels 1-4 Course

2010   The Essence Of Sound,
ISBN 978-0-973854-2-7

Chakra Workshop

Neuro-linguistic programming (NLP) is an approach to communication, personal development, and psychotherapy created by Richard Bandler and John Grinder in California, United States in the 1970s.

Orca Institute

2007   Counseling Hypnotherapist Course

Quantum University

2019   Quantum Doctor Courses

Segal, Inna

2010   The Secret Language of Your Body ISBN 978-158270-260-5

Thie, John

1973   Touch For Health, ISBN 0-87-516-180-4

Tirtha, Swami Sada Shiva

1998   The Ayurveda Encyclopedia ISBN 0-9658042-2-4

Zeck, Robbi

Aromatic Kinesiology Course

Craig, Greg

Emotional Freedom Techniques (EFT)

Message From The Author

It has been forty years, and I still love hypnotherapy. I love the feeling of being in a trance, and all the mind can see.

If you ever get the chance to be hypnotized by a professional, go, and have a session. It can be one of the most transformational experiences that you can have.

Remember that you can remember almost everything you experienced while in a trance, hear sounds, feel like you are awake, and think to yourself while you are in a trance. The most significant difference will be how you can focus on one thought and change it however you like. It is like watching a movie on your phone compared to a high-definition big-screen T.V.

Shift happens... Create magic!

Dr. Santego

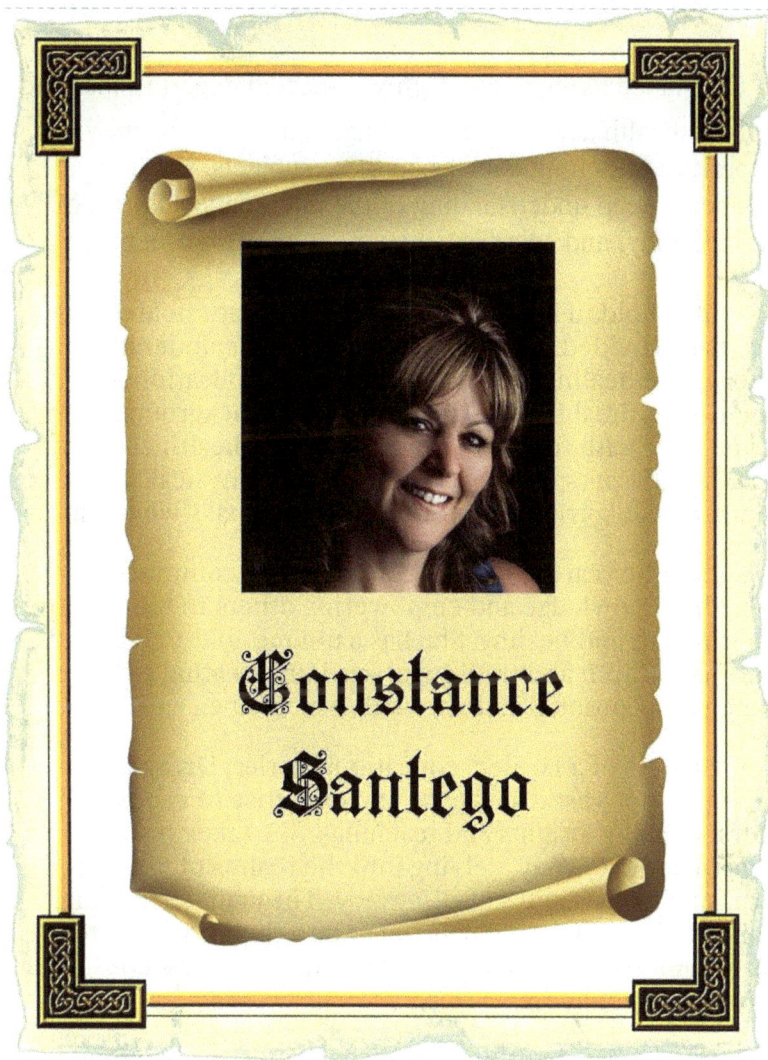

Constance Santego

Shift happens...Create magic!
Dream BIGGER!

Dr. Constance Santego is a highly respected expert in the field of holistic health and spiritual healing. With over twenty years of experience teaching courses on these subjects, she has developed a deep understanding of the interconnectedness of the mind, body, and spirit in achieving overall well-being.

Dr. Santego holds a Ph.D. and Doctorate in Natural Medicine, which has provided her with a comprehensive understanding of alternative healing modalities and their application in promoting optimal health. Her educational background has equipped her with the knowledge to address health concerns from a holistic perspective, considering the physical, emotional, and spiritual aspects of an individual's well-being.

Throughout her career, Dr. Santego has been committed to sharing her knowledge and empowering others to take control of their health and healing. She has a unique ability to blend scientific research and traditional wisdom, creating a bridge between conventional and alternative medicine.

In her "Secrets of a Healer" educational series, Dr. Santego draws upon her vast experience and expertise to captivate readers with her insights and teachings. She takes readers on a transformative journey, delving into the realms of holistic health, spirituality, and self-discovery. Through her writing, she aims to inspire individuals to tap into their own innate healing abilities and embrace a balanced and harmonious approach to well-being.

Dr. Santego's work has touched the lives of many, guiding them toward a more profound understanding of themselves and their connection to the world around them. Her series serves as a beacon of wisdom, offering practical tools and techniques for personal growth and transformation.

Overall, Dr. Constance Santego's blend of knowledge, experience, and passion makes her a captivating figure in the field of holistic health and spiritual healing. Her contributions through teaching, writing, and her spellbinding series continue to inspire and empower individuals on their journeys toward well-being and self-discovery.

ALSO AVAILABLE

Play the game *Ikona* – Discover Your Inner Genie

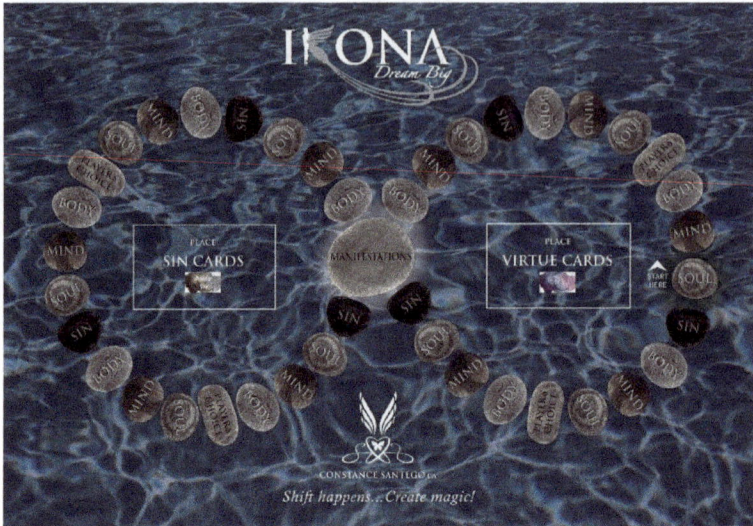

For additional information on

Constance Santego's

wide range of Motivational Products, Coaching Sessions,
Spiritual Retreats,
Live Events and Educational Programs

Go to

www.ConstanceSantego.ca

Follow on Instagram - Constance_Santego and
Facebook - constancesantegoo

Subscribe and receive Free Information and Meditations
on my
YouTube Channel - Constance Santego

www.ingramcontent.com/pod-product-compliance
Lightning Source LLC
Chambersburg PA
CBHW072120020426
42334CB00018B/1658